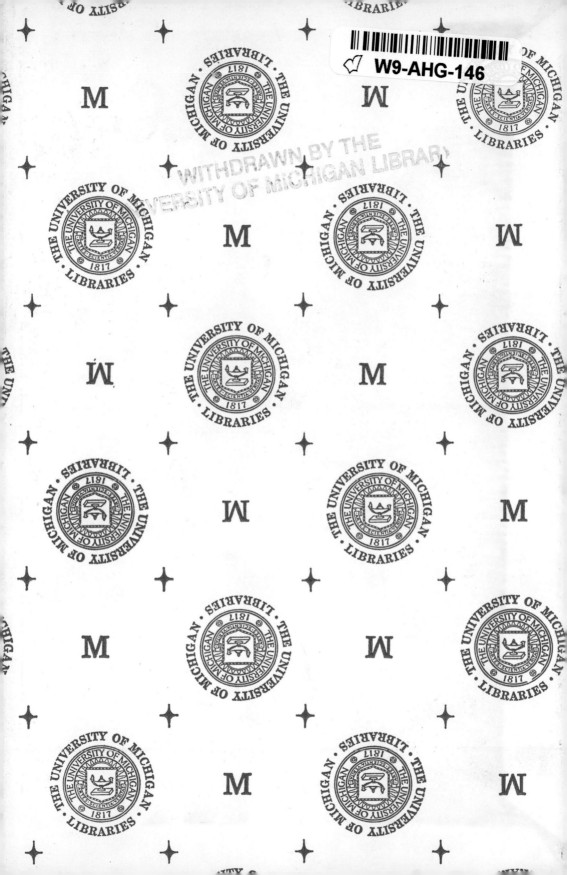

PATIENT CARE STUDIES IN
MEDICAL-SURGICAL NURSING

Patient care studies in
Medical-Surgical Nursing

EDITED BY

■ **WILMA J. PHIPPS, R.N., A.M.**

Associate Professor and Chairman of Medical and
Surgical Nursing, Frances Payne Bolton School of
Nursing, Case Western Reserve University; Director
of Medical and Surgical Nursing, University
Hospitals of Cleveland, Cleveland, Ohio

■ **ROSEMARY RICH, R.N., Ph.D.**

Associate Professor of Medical and Surgical Nursing,
Frances Payne Bolton School of Nursing, Case Western
Reserve University, Cleveland, Ohio

The C. V. Mosby Company
SAINT LOUIS   1972

▪ Contributors

JEANETTE BALDWIN, R.N., M.S.N.

Assistant Clinical Professor of Medical and Surgical Nursing, Frances Payne Bolton School of Nursing, Case Western Reserve University; Assistant Director of Medical and Surgical Nursing, University Hospitals of Cleveland

FRANCES R. BROWN, R.N., M.S.N.

Clinical Instructor of Medical and Surgical Nursing, Frances Payne Bolton School of Nursing, Case Western Reserve University; Nurse Clinician, University Hospitals of Cleveland

PATRICIA S. BUERGIN, R.N., B.S.N.

Senior Clinical Nurse, University Hospitals of Cleveland

MARY E. BUSHONG, R.N., M.S.N.

Assistant Clinical Professor of Operating and Recovery Room Nursing, Frances Payne Bolton School of Nursing, Case Western Reserve University; Nurse Clinician, University Hospitals of Cleveland

RUTH BUTLER, R.N., B.S.

Clinical Nurse, University Hospitals of Cleveland

BARBARA J. DALY, R.N., B.S.

Candidate for M.S.N. Degree in Medical and Surgical Nursing, Frances Payne Bolton School of Nursing, Case Western Reserve University, Cleveland

ELLEN HILE DAUGHERTY, R.N., B.S.

Former Senior Clinical Nurse, University Hospitals of Cleveland

CAROLYN BINGHAM DAVIS, R.N., M.S.

Formerly Assistant Clinical Professor of Medical and Surgical Nursing, Frances Payne Bolton School of Nursing, Case Western Reserve University; Nurse Clinician, University Hospitals of Cleveland

ROXIE FERNELIUS, R.N., B.S.N.

Assistant Instructor, College of Nursing, Wayne State University, Detroit, Michigan

NANCY GORENSHEK, R.N., M.S.N.

Clinical Instructor of Medical and Surgical Nursing, Frances Payne Bolton School of Nursing, Case Western Reserve University; Assistant Director of Medical and Surgical Nursing, University Hospitals of Cleveland

JEAN HANYAK, R.N., B.S.N.

Candidate for M.S.N. Degree in Medical and Surgical Nursing, Frances Payne Bolton School of Nursing, Case Western Reserve University, Cleveland

GLORIA A. HENDERSON, R.N., M.S.N.

Instructor of Medical-Surgical Nursing, College of Nursing, University of Illinois at the Medical Center, Chicago, Illinois

MARILYN J. HOWE, R.N., M.S.N.

Assistant Professor of Gynecologic Nursing, Frances Payne Bolton School of Nursing, Case Western Reserve University; Nurse Clinician, University Hospitals of Cleveland

DONNA J. KUKLO, R.N., M.S.N.

Formerly Assistant Professor of Medical and Surgical Nursing, Frances Payne Bolton School of Nursing, Case Western Reserve University, Cleveland

DOROTHY M. LANUZA, R.N., B.S.N.

Candidate for M.S.N. Degree in Medical-Surgical Nursing, College of Nursing, University of Illinois at the Medical Center, Chicago, Illinois

CAROL MITTEN, R.N., M.S.N.

Clinical Instructor of Medical and Surgical Nursing, Frances Payne Bolton School of Nursing, Case Western Reserve University; Nurse Clinician, University Hospitals of Cleveland

ELAINE NICHOLS, R.N., M.S.N.

Retired

MARGARET A. PALERMO, R.N., M.S.N.

Instructor of Medical and Surgical Nursing, Frances Payne Bolton School of Nursing, Case Western Reserve University, Cleveland

WILMA J. PHIPPS, R.N., A.M.

Associate Professor and Chairman of Medical and Surgical Nursing, Frances Payne Bolton School of Nursing, Case Western Reserve University; Director of Medical and Surgical Nursing, University Hospitals of Cleveland

ELIZABETH FORD PITORAK, R.N., M.S.N.

Associate Professor of Medical and Surgical Nursing, Frances Payne Bolton School of Nursing, Case Western Reserve University, Cleveland

ROSEMARY RICH, R.N., Ph.D.

Associate Professor of Medical and Surgical Nursing, Frances Payne Bolton School of Nursing, Case Western Reserve University, Cleveland

MARJORIE ROTT, R.N., M.S.N.

Instructor of Medical and Surgical Nursing, Frances Payne Bolton School of Nursing, Case Western Reserve University, Cleveland

SANDRA S. SHUMWAY, R.N., M.S.N.

Director of Nursing Care, Hough Norwood Family Center, Cleveland

ARDITH SUDDUTH, R.N., M.S.N.

Assistant Professor of Medical and Surgical Nursing, Frances Payne Bolton School of Nursing, Case Western Reserve University, Cleveland

GAYLE TRAVER, R.N., M.S.N.

Instructor of Internal Medicine, College of Medicine; Assistant Professor, College of Nursing, University of Arizona, Tucson, Arizona

JEAN WILLACKER, R.N., M.S.N.

Clinical Instructor of Medical and Surgical Nursing, Frances Payne Bolton School of Nursing, Case Western Reserve University; Nurse Clinician, University Hospitals of Cleveland

▪ Preface

Nurses working in all types of settings (hospitals, public health agencies, etc.) are constantly being asked to assess patients in terms of their nursing needs and to plan care to meet these needs. In an attempt to help nurses see how assessment and nursing intervention might be planned, we have gathered together in this book a series of care studies.

You will note that the studies vary in approach and in format, but that each one addresses itself to the needs of a particular patient and the nursing actions taken to meet these needs. It is our hope that they will help both nursing students and practicing nurses to apply the nursing process as they care for patients.

Although the studies can be used to supplement any medical-surgical text, some readers of Shafer's *Medical-Surgical Nursing** have expressed a desire to have care study material available to them, therefore these studies are arranged so that they can be used in conjunction with that book. A chart showing the care studies that are relevant to the chapters in *Medical-Surgical Nursing* can be found in the appendix.

Wilma J. Phipps ▪ Rosemary Rich

---

*Shafer, Kathleen N., Sawyer, Janet R., McCluskey, Audrey M., Beck, Edna L., and Phipps, Wilma J.: Medical-Surgical Nursing, ed. 5, St. Louis, 1971, The C. V. Mosby Co.

■ Contents

PATIENT CARE STUDIES IN
MEDICAL-SURGICAL NURSING

CHAPTER 1

PSYCHOSOCIAL PROBLEMS OF A WOMAN WITH MAJOR ALTERATION IN APPEARANCE

BARBARA J. DALY

MEDICAL HISTORY

Miss Green, a 54-year-old secretary was admitted to the hospital on August 8. Miss Green's chief complaints were hearing loss in and discharge from the right ear and paralysis of the right lower eyelid. Miss Green also had multiple skin lesions that she said had increased in number over the past 15 years. Five years ago the lesions were diagnosed as basal cell carcinoma, and she was hospitalized at that time for treatment of the lesions by electrodesiccation, radiation, and excision. Miss Green came to the hospital now expecting to have two operations: one for removal of a tumor from her ear, which would involve a partial or total amputation of the ear, and subsequent plastic surgery to reconstruct the ear.

Over a period of 4 months she underwent seven operations, which resulted in marked alteration of her appearance. Although Miss Green had numerous physical needs throughout her hospitalization, the type and extent of the surgery created special psychologic and social problems for her. Therefore, this study focuses on Miss Green's behavior and emotional needs and the nursing intervention that was used to meet these needs.

PSYCHOSOCIAL BACKGROUND

Miss Green, an only child, lived with her parents until their deaths. She completed high school, but it was not until 5 years later, after the sudden death of her father, that she obtained employment as a secretary in a firm where she continued to work for 29 years. Her mother, who suffered a series of strokes, became progressively weaker and disoriented and was unable to care for herself. Miss Green supported and took care of her mother until her mother's death 13 years ago. Since that time, she has lived alone. Miss Green has one married cousin living in a nearby state but no close relatives.

TREATMENT

The surgery proved to be more extensive than Miss Green had anticipated and the following operations were performed:

1. Total amputation of the right ear on August 12; a split-thickness graft taken from the right thigh was placed over the temporal area
2. Additional repair of the temporal site by a split-thickness graft taken from the right thigh on August 27
3. Excision of a scalp tumor on September 2, at which time her entire head was shaved
4. Exploratory tympanotomy on September 14 in preparation for a temporal bone resection
5. Temporal bone resection on September 25 and pedicle flap rotated from the shoulder to cover the temporal area; a skin graft from the right thigh was placed over the shoulder
6. Another graft to cover the shoulder on October 6, along with a right tarsorrhaphy to correct the paralysis of the lower eyelid
7. Exploratory laparotomy on October 27, as well as a cholecystectomy and a right pyelolithotomy

On the day of the sixth operation, Miss Green developed epigastric distress, which she identified as "gas pain." The pain increased in severity and was not relieved by change in diet, by modification of activity, or by the use of narcotics. Meperidine HCl (Demerol) was increased from 50 mg. intramuscularly every 4 hours p.r.n. to 100 mg. In addition, 25 mg. of hydroxyzine HCl (Vistaril) was ordered every 2 hours p.r.n. An upper gastrointestinal series, small-bowel series, and barium enema were negative. However, a flat plate of the abdomen revealed a large right renal calculus, and a cholecystogram indicated a large stone in the gallbladder. A retrograde pyelogram confirmed right renal lithiasis with obstruction at the pyeloureteral junction, hydronephrosis, and marked cortical thinning of the right kidney. Because Miss Green's symptoms were not typical of either biliary or renal colic, the laparotomy was considered necessary. Exploration confirmed the preoperative diagnoses and also revealed pancreatitis of the uncinate lobe; palpation revealed no other abdominal lesions. A cholecystectomy and right renal lithotomy were performed; Miss Green tolerated these procedures well and returned to her room with a nasogastric tube in place.

NURSING GOALS AND INTERVENTIONS

The needs and nursing care objectives for Miss Green changed considerably from the time of her first surgery until her discharge 4 months later. Each successive operation resulted in further alteration of her appearance—amputation of the ear, shaving of her head, removal of the temporal bone (which resulted in right-sided facial paralysis), and removal of skin from many donor sites for grafts (which resulted in scars)—all undoubtedly had an effect on how Miss Green perceived herself. Because she seemed to demonstrate several distinct conflicts at different stages of her illness, the aspects of her care relating to her behavior required frequent modifications.

The nursing objectives in physical care included measures to promote healing of the skin grafts. Thus pressure dressings were maintained to prevent fluid accumulation, and Miss Green was kept off the side that had been operated upon. She was reminded not to blow her nose, because pressure could be deflected through the eustachian tube to the operative site and could disrupt the graft. Since she had a mild urinary tract infection upon admission, she was treated with acetyl sulfisoxazole (Gantrisin) and acetic acid bladder irrigations, and was encouraged to take fluids, such as prune and cranberry juices, that would provide for an acid pH of the urine.

Until the time of the temporal bone resection, Miss Green, at least overtly, seemed to be coping well with the surgical interventions. She was consistently cheerful and optimistic and spent much time out of her room visiting with other patients. She expressed gratitude for the successful operations and verbalized faith in her doctors and confidence that she would recover. She appreciated the nursing staff and said that she liked everyone except for one nurse with whom she had argued. Although she did not actively practice any formal religion, she had faith in God and believed that He would take care of her and that things would work out for the best. She seemed to have an accurate and realistic understanding of what was involved in the resection, although she did postpone this decision. She did not directly refer to any alteration in her appearance, but was aware of the facial nerve involvement and indicated a need to talk over the recommendation that she have the temporal bone resection.

Initially, time was spent giving her factual information and answering questions. Later, she was encouraged to talk over these facts and to express any concerns about the operation. She verbalized fear that she might incur brain damage, but seemed reassured when told that the tumor did not involve any brain structures and that the operation would not alter her intellectual abilities.

After Miss Green had the temporal bone resection, several changes became evident in her behavior. Although she appeared cheerful, this affect was put forth with some effort. Her talk of faith, in both doctors and God, decreased considerably. She expressed anger toward the night nursing staff for such things as not answering her call light soon enough and for delaying medications. She did not seem to obtain any relief from verbalizing these complaints; she repeated them over and over. Her use of denial and projection was identified: she avoided looking in the mirror and refused to see or talk to friends, saying that her appearance and slurred speech would upset them.

The nursing objectives at this time were to support Miss Green and help her express her anger and to explore the extent of denial by allowing, but not supporting it. It was questioned whether the staff was the real and sole cause of her anger, or whether the anger was a reflection of her feelings about all that had happened to her. She expressed no feelings directly related to the surgery and the subsequent alteration in her appearance. Although she seemed appreciative of the opportunity to talk, this apparently did not alter either the need to verbalize or the intensity of feeling. With the exception of recognizing her difficulty in eating and speaking, Miss Green did not refer to any feelings she herself had about her appearance. The significance of the facial alteration, as expressed by her, seemed to lie only in the changes in functional ability and the impact of her appearance upon others. For example, although she recognized an interference in the ability to ingest food, she denied any feelings about this interference.

The rationale suggesting the kind of emotional support Miss Green needed at this time was that her use of projection and denial were probably acting as necessary helping mechanisms in coping with the changes brought about by surgery. These defenses may have been allowing her to reduce the impact of the surgery until she had the opportunity to recognize that she was still accepted and liked by those around her despite her appearance. For this reason, no attempt was made to challenge her denial or to force conversation about her own feelings at this point, and no attempt was made to have her look at herself in a mirror.

Miss Green returned from the temporal bone surgery with a large pressure dressing over her head and right shoulder; her right arm was strapped to her chest. Because of this forced position and because the skin grafts were taken from the back of her thigh, she had more discomfort than previously; thus the focus was on providing physical comfort. Analgesics were used frequently, her position was altered often, and her thigh dressing was changed frequently. The edema and paralysis of the right side of her face made chewing, drinking, and swallowing difficult, and since she could not feed herself at first, another objective was to maintain adequate oral intake. Soft foods and liquids were served and fed slowly, frequent snacks and her favorite juices and soft drinks were given throughout the day, and ice chips were kept by her bedside.

Two weeks after the temporal bone resection, Miss Green had had her final skin graft, and all operative areas were healing well. Her intake was adequate, no infection was present, and she was ambulating well, although abdominal pain was beginning at this time. Her use of denial continued: she obviously avoided looking in mirrors, refused to wash her own face, and remained in her room during the day with her chair turned so that the operative side was away from the door. She was probably still using projection when she spoke of the feelings, the difficulties, and stress of another patient who had undergone a mandibulectomy. She continued to express anger, now also directed at the intern caring for her. The repetitiveness increased to the point of repeating incidents and complaints word for word. She also tried to exert a measure of control by insisting that certain things be done at certain times. She spoke of the changes brought about by her talking to her doctor about the night staff—in effect, the control she exerted.

Miss Green initially came to the hospital expecting only to undergo two operations. Instead, she was subjected to seven surgical episodes, which resulted in prolonged hospitalization and a life-threatening diagnosis requiring a difficult decision and adjustment to a gross alteration of her appearance. The rationale influencing the kind of response that was indicated, therefore, was that she needed to believe that she could bring about changes in her environment and could control, at least to some extent, what was happening to her. This belief in herself may have been imperative for Miss Green, who lived alone and was accustomed to having total control over her life. Therefore, the nurse allowed her to direct much of her own care and verbally recognized her reports of control over other staff members, such as the changes she brought about by insisting on having things done in a certain way. Miss Green was allowed to make as many decisions as possible concerning diet, bath, and time of changing dressings, and her response to this decision-making was favorable.

Another objective at this time was to attempt to help Miss Green focus her anger directly on the source. It was thought that unless she could obtain some relief through expressing her anger, she might begin to turn it inward and become depressed. Attempts were made to determine whether some of her anger might be appropriately related to either the surgeon or perhaps the surgical insult itself, but Miss Green did not respond to leading questions and never expressed any feelings about all that had happened to her. The nurse continued to provide opportunities for her to express anger, however, and attempted to show her that anger is an acceptable mode of behavior. Although her denial was not verbally confronted, the nurse directed some actions toward minimizing the degree to which this denial governed Miss Green's behavior. For example, Miss Green was reassured that she would not dislodge her dressings and was encouraged to wash her own face. She was encouraged to ambulate in the hall rather than in her room. In addition, the possibility of wearing a wig until her hair grew out was discussed.

As Miss Green's abdominal pain grew more severe, physical and emotional needs began to merge. She was apprehensive about the cause of her pain and required a great deal of reassurance as well as frequent use of analgesics. She also seemed to have some fear that the staff would think her pain was "imagined," and this fear may have been an accurate reflection of some staff members' feelings. Prior to the laparotomy, objectives for her care focused upon observation of what factors might be influencing the onset of pain, explaining the laboratory and X-ray results to her, and explaining nursing actions such as the straining of urine for renal calculi. Miss Green seemed to receive some reassurance by gaining understanding of these things; thus an effort was made to provide the factual information she needed. Expressions of belief in and recognition of her pain and the physiologic cause of it were repeatedly made.

After her abdominal surgery, Miss Green remained in considerable discomfort. Much of the discomfort was caused by the nasogastric tube and intravenous infusions, which frequently infiltrated and needed to be restarted. Her need for narcotics continued, and there was some concern that she was becoming addicted to meperidine. Faced with this possibility, Miss Green responded as though she thought the staff did not believe the pain was real. She did seem, at times, to request the meperidine sooner than necessary, possibly because she feared she would not get the medication when she needed it later. The nurse again attempted to convey to Miss Green her recognition of the reality of the pain and to provide the analgesic when requested. The objective was twofold: to reduce anxiety, which may have been a contributing cause of the pain, and to provide reassurance that Miss Green would receive medication upon request so that she would feel free to lengthen the time between doses.

The issue of exerting control was still evident, for Miss Green became even more adamant about deciding when she would eat, sleep, and ambulate. The staff, concerned about the length of time she remained in bed, encouraged her to ambulate. Miss Green strongly refused to comply with their wishes. The objective was to ambulate the patient, but by use of the rationale that Miss Green would act according to her need to exert some control over her environment and daily schedule, the appropriate action was to present her with a series of alternatives that included the objective, but left some choice. For example, rather than telling her that she should eat breakfast, then have her bath, and then walk the length of the hall, she was asked whether she wanted to eat before or after her bath, whether she wanted to walk before or after her bath, and how far she thought she could walk that day. She responded positively to this technique and slowly progressed.

As the date for discharge grew nearer, Miss Green expressed anxiety about caring for herself at home. She had been hospitalized for a period of 4 months, and it seemed probable that physical care was not her only concern. Physical deformity is threatening to anyone, and Miss Green's reactions to her change in appearance have already been discussed; however, deformities are far more acceptable in the hospital environment than in a patient's normal life setting. Also, Miss Green had become accustomed to being dependent and to never being alone; now she was to return to an empty apartment. These aspects as a cause of anxiety were suggested to Miss Green, but she denied them almost completely and identified only concerns about who would cook and help her with her bath and where she would get her medications.

As a final nursing measure, plans were made and discussed with Miss Green before discharge for the nurse who cared for her throughout her illness to visit her at home several times to help make the transition from the hospital to the home environment. A referral was also made to the Visiting Nurse Agency in an attempt to provide a helping person outside the hospital who could assist Miss Green in coping with the adjustment of living at home with her altered appearance.

CHAPTER 2

PROVIDING COMFORT FOR AN ELDERLY MAN DURING HIS TERMINAL ILLNESS

ARDITH SUDDUTH

MEDICAL HISTORY

Mr. Hank Johns, an 85-year-old white male, was admitted to the hospital for a diagnostic evaluation after complaints of weakness, nausea, and anorexia for 3 weeks prior to admission. For the several weeks before admission, he had experienced constipation and irregularity of bowel habits. Three years prior to admission he had a colectomy for a cancer of the colon. Three months prior to admission he had a cataract removed from the left eye. After a medical evaluation the diagnosis of metastatic cancer of the liver was made. The medical and nursing care goals were palliative measures to promote rest and comfort until his death, which occurred 3 weeks after admission. Although his condition deteriorated steadily, he remained pain free, requiring increasing amounts of physical care.

PSYCHOSOCIAL BACKGROUND

Mr. Johns was a retired vice president of a small tool company. He owned his own home in a fashionable suburb and lived with his confused, senile wife until 3 weeks prior to his admission when she was admitted with a fractured hip. He had Medicare, health insurance, and adequate savings to cover the costs of his medical care. He and his wife had engaged a full-time housekeeper and nurse to assist them in managing their own care and the care of the home.

The couple had three children, all married with families. One daughter and her family live in the city and visited her mother and father daily. Mr. Johns was an Episcopalian and had been an active church member until about 1 year before his death; his priest visited often during his illness.

Mr. Johns was admitted to a private room next to his wife, but she was discharged 2 weeks later to enter an extended care facility. Throughout the mutual hospitalization, Mr. Johns visited his wife twice daily in the afternoons and evenings. During these visits, Mrs. Johns seemed to become more alert and rational when Mr. Johns talked and planned for their future. He discussed with her the plans for her placement in an extended care facility and told her that he did not think they would ever live at their own home together again. Although he knew he was gravely ill, he tried to keep a cheerful, well appearance before his wife. He rarely used the words dying or death, but spoke occasionally about how he had his affairs in order and that he would "never leave this place alive." It appeared to the nurse that he was preparing for his death, and during his hospitalization he withdrew more and more from the busy activities of the world. He gave the impression that he indeed accepted the inevitability of death and was ready.

TREATMENT
Medical orders

Darvon Compound, 65 mg., p.r.n. for pain.
Colace, 50 mg., every morning.
Daily vital signs.
1500 mg. of sodium, high-protein diet.

Diagnostic studies

Liver scan—abnormal; large with superoinferior diameter of right lobe about 28 cm. and transverse diameter about 23 cm.; multiple areas of space-occupying lesions possibly a result of metastases.
I.V. cholangiogram—within normal limits.
Barium enema—primary cancer of the colon (splenic flexure) about 7 cm. in length narrowed to less than 1 cm.; hepatic flexure displaced downward to the region of the iliac crest.
Upper gastrointestinal series—normal stomach and duodenum; stomach displaced to the left by a large left lobe of the liver.

Laboratory studies

TESTS	AT ADMISSION	1 WEEK AFTER ADMISSION	NORMAL VALUES
Blood urea nitrogen	46	60	10-20 mg./100 ml.
Fasting glucose	75	65	65-110 mg./100 ml.
Sodium	132	129	134-145 mEq./L.
Potassium	4.7	5.1	3.5-5 mEq./L.
CO_2 (content)	27		25-32 mM./L.
Red blood count	3.37	3.26	4.6-6.2 million/mm.[3]
Hematocrit	34.7	34.1	40-54 vol.%
White blood count	16,200	18,200	4800-10,800 mm.[3]

Guaiac—stool positive for occult blood

NURSING CARE PLAN

DATA	OBJECTIVES	NURSING INTERVENTIONS
An aged, gravely ill man for whom death is imminent.	Provide dignity and respect during terminal illness. Provide comfort and rest. Plan visiting with hospitalized wife.	These two major objectives permeated all care given to Mr. Johns during his hospitalization. Consult with wife's nurse to coordinate her care so that she is ready for husband's visit.
Likes to visit wife at 2:00 P.M. and 7:00 P.M.		
Becoming progressively weaker and requiring more and more assistance with dressing and walking.		Assist Mr. Johns with getting robe and slippers on as necessary. Take to visit wife in wheelchair at 2:00 P.M. and 7:00 P.M.
Usually visits only 15 to 20 min. Prefers to have nurse ask him if he is ready to go rather than for him to ask to leave his wife. Daughter visits about 8:00 P.M.; Mr. Johns appreciates her visits.		Check back at 2:15 and 7:15 to see if he is ready to go back to own room. Help him back to bed for rest period.
Seldom wishes to discuss his illness. Occasionally initiates conversation by saying, "I'm very ill. My wife is confused and I don't want to worry her."	Allow opportunity to discuss his care and death.	Listen to what Mr. Johns has to say.
Daughter concerned about her father; asks about his condition; reassured by information about care her father is getting.	Support daughter.	Listen to daughter. Volunteer information about father's care such as foods being offered, assistance being given. Be sure Mr. Johns is rested and positioned comfortably before visitors arrive.
Minister visits about 10:00 A.M. for approximately 5 min.; Mr. Johns seems to appreciate these visits very much.		Plan care so Mr. Johns will not be disturbed while seeing minister.

NURSING CARE PLAN—cont'd

DATA	OBJECTIVES	NURSING INTERVENTIONS
Throughout hospitalization until last 3 days of life, desired to be kept aware of current events through daily morning newspaper.	Meet needs of keeping in contact with the outside world.	Buy daily newspaper from newsboy with money kept in bedside drawer for this purpose.
Does not like newspaper read to him.		
Hard of hearing.		
Hearing-aid glasses kept in bedside table.	Provide assistance when needed to maintain supportive aids.	Assist with cleaning glasses and magnifying glass with specially treated papers in bedside table prior to reading newspaper.
Hearing-aid glasses uncomfortable to lie on; therefore, removes them except for visitors.		
Lip-reads.	Provide verbal communication, which Mr. Johns can "hear."	Face Mr. Johns when speaking; speak slowly and clearly; get his attention before speaking.
Decreased vision.		Will respond to verbal stimuli of moderate tone when he sees person at a distance of approximately 3 feet.
Wears second pair of glasses without hearing aid.		
Takes off glasses when he wishes to sleep or to be undisturbed.	Allow to withdraw from world as he wishes.	Provide quiet, calm environment at times determined by Mr. Johns.
Skin dry.	Maintain intact integumentum.	Use 2 capfuls bath oil in bath water.
Skin turgor doughy, 2 to 3+ pitting edema of feet and legs to the knees.		No soap on skin.
		Apply lotion generously to arms and legs.
		Apply elastic stockings, large size; remove at least b.i.d. and give skin care (9:00 A.M., before bath; 8:00 P.M., prior to evening care); every M., W., F., apply clean pair of elastic stockings after bath.
		Passive range of motion to joints during bath as tolerated.

Continued.

NURSING CARE PLAN—cont'd

DATA	OBJECTIVES	NURSING INTERVENTIONS
Likes to wear sponge-rubber elbow protectors.		Remove elbow protectors 9:00 A.M., 8:00 P.M., and p.r.n. at Mr. Johns' wish; apply lotion to elbows with gentle stimulating motion.
Nearly totally independent on admission; became progressively dependent on nursing staff for meeting physical needs.		Sheepskin under him from shoulders to hips. Help him change position; turn side to back to side.
Large abdominal mass, especially on right side.		Position of comfort is left side, bed flat, one small pillow under head.
Early in care, up in chair for meals.		Up in padded lounge chair as tolerated.
Gradually spent more time in bed.		Pin call light to gown.
Up twice a day until day before his death.		Check every 10 min. to see if ready to go to bed.
Mr. Johns' one major request during his entire hospitalization was to be shaved with his straightedge razor early in the morning before physician rounds about 10:00 A.M.	Assist with personal hygiene.	Assemble shaving equipment on overbed table: basin of hot water, aerosol shaving cream, straightedge razor. Place mirror so he can see. Assist with shaving as necessary.
Last week of illness, requested nurse to shave him.		Uses aftershave lotion kept in bedside table.
Bad taste in mouth. Appetite poor. Own teeth in good repair.		Brushes teeth on arising and after meals: 8:00 A.M., 9:00 A.M., 1:00 P.M., 6:00 P.M. Offer mouthwash prior to meals (12:00 noon and 5:00 P.M.) and at h.s.
Nutritional intake decreased over entire hospitalization.	Maintain food and fluid intake to meet metabolic needs.	Offer fluids q.1h. during day, 8:00 A.M. to 8:00 P.M.

NURSING CARE PLAN—cont'd

DATA	OBJECTIVES	NURSING INTERVENTIONS
Fluid intake 700 ml. on most days.		Help him make out menu each morning; help choose soft, nutritious foods and fluids in small amounts.
Abdominal mass gave feeling of fullness continuously.		
Likes cold liquids, especially orange juice, iced tea, and hot cereal for breakfast.		Offer supplemental foods between meals and at h.s.: 10:00 A.M., 3:00 P.M., and 8:00 P.M.
Urinary output decreased over hospitalization.	Monitor intake and output.	Record intake and output each shift.
		Assist on and off bedside commode for bowel movement, usually after breakfast.
Does not ask to have urinal emptied.		Check urinal q.1h. to be sure empty.
		Replace in bed with Mr. Johns.

Three weeks after Mr. Johns was admitted, he died quietly in his sleep about 6:00 A.M. During the last 24 hours of his life, he required total nursing care. He was not fully responsive and was very weak. He was shaved lying nearly flat in bed. Unable to take fluids, his mouth was moistened often with cotton swabs soaked in a diluted mouthwash solution. Mr. Johns said little, but expressed his appreciation of the comfort measures with his eyes. The evening before he died, his daughter visited him and he recognized her. She sat quietly in the room awhile and told him his wife was doing well, and he dozed off. They both seemed to know his death was imminent, and they responded to this knowledge in a quiet, calm manner. The nursing staff felt that they had planned for and met his needs physically and emotionally, and they were glad that they had been able to provide him with care that allowed him to spend his last days in dignity.

NURSING NEEDS OF A WOMAN WITH ALCOHOLISM, CIRRHOSIS, AND DELIRIUM TREMENS

JEAN WILLACKER

MEDICAL AND SOCIAL HISTORY

Mrs. Porter is a 39-year-old housewife and mother of three children, two of whom are teen-agers. She was a barmaid for 10 years and, at present, she and her husband own a delicatessen. Both she and her husband have a problem with alcohol.

Mrs. Porter has a history of cirrhosis for which she has been followed in the clinic. She recently developed ascites and 3+ pitting edema of the legs. During her visits to the clinic, medical and nursing personnel have worked with her in an effort to help her stay away from alcohol. Throughout this period, her husband has refused to visit the clinic and denied that he has any difficulty with alcohol. While preparing food one day, Mrs. Porter spilled boiling water on her foot. She said that she had had a few beers and her gait was a little unsteady. She suffered a second-degree burn of her right foot, and little healing took place. It was then that she was admitted to the hospital.

The hospitalization, according to Mrs. Porter's viewpoint, helped her escape from family discord and gave her liver a chance to regenerate. Three days after admission, however, she went into delirium tremens. At this time, she began having auditory and visual hallucinations and needed to be restrained. She described her hallucinations as seashells that had the heads of her children and shells for bodies. The seashells were marching into the sea and screaming, "Help us, help us!"

TREATMENT
Laboratory findings

Microcytic hypochromic anemia was treated with folic acid, 5 mg. daily, and ferrous sulfate, 300 mg. t.i.d.

Prothrombin time, 40%—vitamin K was given daily to prevent bleeding.

NURSING CARE PLAN

OBJECTIVES	APPROACH
Protect from injury.	Place in soft restraints; keep on side to prevent aspiration should vomiting occur.
	Give vitamin K as ordered.
Reduce fright.	Have someone stay with Mrs. Porter constantly.
	Keep room quiet and darkened to reduce sensory stimuli.
	Give sedation (chlordiazepoxide [Librium] and paraldehyde) as necessary.
Orient to reality.	When Mrs. Porter hallucinates, bring her back to reality by orienting her to time, place, and person: speak softly and tell her where she is, what time it is, and who is with her. Keep calendar and clock in room.
Provide adequate nutrition.	Add vitamins as ordered to I.V. fluids; maintain I.V. fluid intake at 1000 ml. in 24 hours.
Reduce ascites and dependent edema.	When patient on oral intake, explain need for 250 mg. sodium diet.
	Make a schedule for dividing Mrs. Porter's oral fluid intake of 1000 ml. over a 24-hour period; be sure fluids are spaced so that she can have some on each shift.
Support Mrs. Porter in her desire to give up alcohol.	Be available to her so that she can discuss her feelings about giving up alcohol.
	Reinforce how well she is doing without alcohol.
	Make plans for her to be followed in the clinic by the same doctor and nurse clinician who saw her in the hospital.
	Give her the phone numbers of personnel she can call at any time she feels that she needs a drink.
Acquaint with community resources.	Tell her about AA and other similar groups.
Assist the family in understanding the problems of alcoholism.	Discuss with her the possibility of the children joining a group such as Al-Ateens where they can get support for themselves and help in understanding the problem of alcoholism.

After discharge, Mrs. Porter joined a group of alcoholic patients who meet weekly in the clinic. The treatment used is called "reality group therapy." Through verbalization in the group, Mrs. Porter is able to see how others face the problem of alcoholism, and the support she receives from the group gives her enough strength to face another week of abstinence. The nurse clinician and the doctor working with Mrs. Porter are trying to get her husband interested in this kind of program. They have also encouraged Mrs. Porter to telephone them whenever she feels anxious about drinking. In addition, the nurse has reminded her about how ill she had been and about how well she feels now in an effort to prevent her from feeling overconfident and thus desirous of drinking again. A chronic problem takes a long time to resolve, and Mrs. Porter understands now that she must always be on guard against the urge to drink. Many impulse drinkers use disulfiram (Antabuse) to curb this urge, but so far it has not been necessary for Mrs. Porter.

CHAPTER 4

A YOUNG MAN WITH CEREBRAL DAMAGE FROM AN ACCIDENT

DOROTHY M. LANUZA

MEDICAL HISTORY

Frank Jones, a 16-year-old male, was in an automobile accident early in January. When brought to the emergency room of Community Hospital he was deeply comatose and was experiencing respiratory difficulty; for several minutes there was some question of cardiac arrest. While he was in the emergency room, an endotracheal tube was inserted and the cuff inflated. Suctioning was carried out to provide an adequate airway. Approximately 450 ml. of gastric contents smelling of alcohol was obtained in this way. It was thought that this material had been aspirated prior to intubation. Although Frank was placed on the Bennett respirator for a short period of time, it was felt that his condition was becoming stabilized and, with suctioning, an adequate airway was maintained; thus a tracheostomy was not necessary at this time. Lacerations in his right temporal and left parietal areas were sutured. The initial diagnosis was "severe general cerebral contusion with scalp lacerations in the right temporal and left parietal areas with possible basilar fracture." When Frank's condition was stable, he was transferred to the intensive care unit.

Upon admission to the intensive care unit, Frank was examined by a neurosurgeon. Blood pressure and pulse were within normal limits. He was in a deep coma with small, but equal, pupils. Eye movements were slightly disconjugate with the right eye exhibiting a slight lateral deviation. He had no spontaneous movement and his lower extremities did not move upon stimulation; however a Babinski response was present. His upper extremities would extend slightly on repeated, deep, painful stimulation. Respirations were much improved. There was no evidence of spinal fluid leak. During a period of approximately 1½ hours, suctioning elicited flexion of his arms and leg movements. At this point, both the emergency room physician and the neurosurgeon agreed that, although Frank's condition was still critical, marked improvement had been made.

The next day, Frank was taken to surgery. Burr holes were made in the skull to treat a subdural hematoma, and a tracheostomy was performed. It was 3 weeks before Frank regained consciousness and slowly began demonstrating improvement in his condition. Speech began to return about 3 months after the initial trauma; 3 weeks later he was transferred to the rehabilitation hospital.

PSYCHOSOCIAL BACKGROUND

Frank's parents are divorced. His mother, who has legal custody of Frank and two younger children, has remarried and is pregnant. She said that Frank seemed generally hostile since her remarriage and that he has rejected his stepfather. Prior to the accident, Frank left his mother and went to live with his father in another community. Frank's mother, Mrs. Green, describes Frank as a dependent, yet very bright boy who did well in school, although he has been under the care of a psychiatrist since shortly after his parents' divorce.

It was noted that when admitted to the hospital immediately after the accident, some alcohol-smelling material was suctioned. When the neurosurgeon met with Frank's mother and stepfather and discussed the boy's critical condition, he mentioned this. At this point, Mrs. Green asked whether there was any evidence of "dope" and wanted to know if the neurosurgeon planned to run any tests for dope. There were no plans to perform such an analysis, and the reason for Mrs. Green's concern about dope is not known.

TREATMENT FOR ACUTE PHASE—patient comatose
Medical therapy
Medications
>   Dexamethasone (Decadron), 0.75 mg., daily.
>   Diphenylhydantoin sodium (Dilantin), 100 mg., t.i.d.
>   Chlordiazepoxide (Librium), 10 mg., t.i.d.
Treatments
>   Insert Foley catheter and irrigate b.i.d. with Solu G solution.
>   Tracheostomy.
>>   Suction p.r.n.
>>   Clean inner cannula q.3h. for first 48 hours, and then b.i.d. and p.r.n.
>>   Change tracheostomy dressing p.r.n.

Diagnostic tests
Skull X-rays—no evidence of fracture.
Chest X-ray—some evidence of aspiration.

Laboratory tests
All laboratory tests were found to be within normal limits.

NURSING CARE PLAN

OBJECTIVE	NURSING INTERVENTION
Maintain an adequate airway.	Position patient on side or in a semiprone position. Suction p.r.n. to remove secretions and prevent obstruction. Employ aseptic technique in suctioning the tracheostomy to prevent infection. Clean inner cannula q.3h. for first 48 hours, and then b.i.d. and p.r.n. Change tracheostomy dressing p.r.n. Prevent drying out of tracheal mucosa by using steam vaporizer p.r.n. Check carefully for cyanosis during first few days.
Give intensive nursing care and observe neurologic status of patient.	Observe and report: 1. Level of consciousness 2. Pupillary size and response 3. Vital signs 4. Motor and sensory function 5. Whether corneal reflex and gag reflex are present 6. When seizures occur; the nurse must (a) insert tongue blade or airway in mouth and (b) carefully observe and record type of seizure 7. Emotional response of patient to stimuli 8. Drainage from any area; particular notice should be taken of otorrhea and rhinorrhea; sterile cotton pledgets are used in orifice with a spinal fluid leak
Maintain adequate fluid and nutritional balance.	**Unconscious state** Observe and accurately record I.V. intake. Gastric feedings: Check to see that tube is in patient's stomach before each feeding to prevent aspiration. 100 to 200 ml. feedings q.2-3h. Flush tube after meal with 50 ml. of water. Change tube q.5d. **Conscious state** Maintain adequate fluid intake. Encourage adequate nutritional intake.
Maintain adequate elimination. Urinary system— Foley catheter. Bowel.	 Keep accurate intake and output record. Follow doctor's orders regarding fluid intake. Maintain asepsis during catheter insertion and irrigation. Begin a basic bowel program to prevent impaction. Doctor may order digital removal of stool daily or rectal suppositories, or possibly enemas q.2-3d.

Continued.

NURSING CARE PLAN—cont'd

OBJECTIVE	NURSING INTERVENTION
Maintain intact integument.	Keep skin clean and massage frequently. Apply lanolin to feet and dry areas. Use alternating air mattress and turn patient q.2h. Keep toenails and fingernails short and clean.
Give mouth care.	Brush teeth twice a day. Clean q.2-4h. with normal saline or alkaline mouthwash solution.
Take care of eyes.	Check several times a day for signs of irritation or for lack of corneal reflex.
Maintain body temperature within normal limits.	Take rectal temperature q.4h. when hyperthermia occurs. Institute measures to lower temperature. Apply extra covering p.r.n. for hypothermia.

TREATMENT FOR CHRONIC PHASE

Almost 4 months after his accident Frank Jones was transferred to the rehabilitation hospital. His diagnosis at this time was "severe traumatic encephalopathy." The results of the physical and neurologic examination contained the following impressions:

1. Diffuse brain damage
2. Right hemiplegia, secondary to brain damage
3. Aphasia, both receptive and expressive, secondary to brain damage
4. Right homonymous hemianopia (blindness in the right half of each eye), secondary to brain damage

Medical therapy

Medications
    Diphenylhydantoin sodium, 100 mg., t.i.d.
    Dexamethasone, 5 mg., daily.
Speech therapy
Physical therapy
Occupational therapy—evaluate with respect to activities of daily living (ADL), prepare to live at home with mother and stepfather, and try ambulation—if not practical, use tilt table.
Social service
Psychology. In evaluating Frank's condition, the psychologist at the rehabilitation hospital stated, "The organic deficits for immediate memory are

real, but personality regression may, in part, be psychogenic and may be related to his premorbid stresses or conflicts."

Laboratory findings

CBC within normal limits.

Chest X-ray film within normal limits.

Brain scan—12.7 millicuries of technetium. Brain scan in four projections shows no abnormal uptake. Conclusion—Normal brain scan.

EEG. The impression is that this record shows moderate degree of abnormality throughout the left side but a maximum on left frontal and left temporal areas, indicating the presence of cerebral damage within those regions. The depression of activity indicates that a subdural type of abnormality cannot be entirely excluded. No epileptiform discharges were seen.

NURSING ASSESSMENT AND INTERVENTION

The nurse as a member of the rehabilitation health team must work closely with the other disciplines, such as occupational therapy, physical therapy, and social service, and, when possible, must try to provide in the nursing care plan application of what the patient is being taught by these disciplines.

Activities of daily living

Dressing and hygiene. Frank can undress and dress upper extremities and do hygiene with step-by-step directions. He needs assistance to dress and undress lower extremities.

Transfer. Frank transfers with the assistance of one person, but has difficulty following through on pivot. He attempts to propel wheelchair with left hand only.

Eating. He feeds himself with left hand. Because of his right hemianopia, the utensils are placed so that he can see them with the left half of each eye. He attempts to monitor himself by asking if he is eating too fast or taking too large a bite. Occasionally, he finger-feeds himself. He needs supervision in eating, and so he has most of his meals on the ward for this reason and for safety. When he is attended in the cafeteria, he is usually not distracted or stimulated by the activity of others.

Diet. Frank has an excellent appetite. His fluid intake is quite adequate.

Bowel. Frank's bowel program consists of being toileted every night with digital stimulation and rectal suppository if necessary. He has shown awareness and has requested to go to the bathroom.

Bladder. He wears an external catheter only while at therapies. A toileting schedule with offering a urinal was not very successful. However, placing Frank on the toilet met with complete success (apparently due to association). Frank is frequently incontinent at night.

Sleep. Frank is somewhat restless, but usually sleeps well at night. He tires during the day and requires rest periods, at which time he is frequently positioned on his abdomen to facilitate extension of his right leg. He can voluntarily do this with verbal cues.

Skin. Frank's skin is generally in good condition with occasional redness over the coccyx.

SOCIAL ADJUSTMENT AND COMMUNICATION

Frank is very friendly and cheerful. He is well liked and gets much attention from the staff. He always attempts to cooperate despite an automatic response of "I can't" or "I don't know how." His speech is rapid and somewhat lacking in inflection. He can usually find the words he wants with verbal cues. Visual cues are most effective when accompanied by verbal cues. His responses are usually appropriate in a general way, but he is unable to retain specifics for any length of time. He responds best to short, simple, concrete phrases. Instructions must be kept short and simple, and frequent repetition is necessary. Frank must be encouraged and given sufficient time to communicate, for his orientation to time and place is very poor.

For safety, a tongue blade is kept in the bedside drawer and Frank should have another one with him at all times.

Frank is impulsive and lacks judgment. Therefore, when he is in a wheelchair, he must be strapped in at all times. He is not to be left unattended in the bathroom, and the side rails of his bed are to be kept up. Because he has right homonymous hemianopia, he should be approached from his left side so that he can see the person coming. The loss of the right half of his visual field makes it difficult for him to judge obstructions such as door jambs on his right.

Although Frank's mother is extremely anxious, she usually controls herself in Frank's presence. She has not accepted his condition and still feels that he will recover completely. Mrs. Green openly verbalizes that Frank was becoming a problem before the accident in that he resented his stepfather and was becoming rebellious. She appears angry about this. Even so, Frank's entire family seem to work well with him currently.

NURSING GOALS

1. Enlist the participation of mother in Frank's care and prepare for him to have a weekend pass. This includes teaching Mrs. Green what is in-

volved in Frank's care with special emphasis on communication skills and safety factors.

2. Emphasize the patient's need for consistency from the staff as well as from Frank's family. Limit these expectations to only one or two areas until accomplished.

3. Attempt to decrease the numerous expectations and approaches from staff and friends.

CHAPTER 5

USE OF PREOPERATIVE INFORMATION TO ALLEVIATE FEAR OF CORRECTIVE SURGERY

PATRICIA S. BUERGIN AND MARY E. BUSHONG

MEDICAL HISTORY

Sr. Anna Marie is a 32-year-old teaching nun who has been a diagnosed rheumatoid arthritic for approximately 4 years. Over this 4-year period she has had progressive narrowing of the joint spaces in both knees. This change has made her knees painful and has limited the motion and weight-bearing ability of the knee joints themselves. Consequently, she has found it increasingly difficult to stand, walk, and teach classes.

After following a conservative medical program (aspirin, hydroxychloroquine sulfate, prednisone, exercise, heat application, and crutch-walking) for this 4-year period, she experienced limited relief of pain, and negligible control had been effected over the progression of the joint disease. Because of her diminished ability to assume teaching responsibilities and other activities of daily living, she was admitted to the hospital for corrective surgery.

NURSING INTERVENTION

Inasmuch as Sr. Anna Marie had been a patient in the same hospital when she was diagnosed, the staff referred to prior nursing notes and began to question behavioral changes. Previously, the patient had been quiet, withdrawn, and extremely concerned for her privacy. Now she was effusive, outgoing, and seemed less overtly concerned about privacy.

During the course of preoperative teaching, it was learned that Sr. Anna Marie had had no previous surgical experiences. When questioned, she quickly and jokingly denied feeling nervous or frightened at the prospect of having an operation. Being aware of the patient's former behavioral patterns as opposed to current ones, the nurse thought that Sr. Anna Marie might be concealing a real fear of anesthesia and surgery. The nurse speculated that the patient might fear a loss of control over what she might say while awakening from anesthesia and a loss of privacy during the time when she would be less in control of her environment. In fact, Sr. Anna Marie did express concerns about saying and doing "un-nunly things as I wake up."

One way the nurse attempted to alleviate what she suspected to be fears of this patient was to ask her whether she would like to talk to a nurse from the recovery room. She suggested to Sr. Anna Marie that she might feel more comfortable if there were a familiar person in that area with whom she could relate. Sr. Anna Marie responded positively and a visit was arranged. Sister questioned the recovery room nurse about how patients behave when waking up from anesthesia and about how she would be assisted if she experienced pain or had "to go to the bathroom." The recovery room nurse answered these questions to Sr. Anna Marie's expressed satisfaction and further reassured her that she would be with her in the recovery room.

Sr. Anna Marie had an uncomplicated recovery from anesthesia. Upon awakening, she remembered the preoperative visit of the recovery room nurse and seemed comforted by the fact that she knew someone in the area. Knowing that she could seek relief from pain, she easily asked for assistance when she was uncomfortable.

On the day after surgery, Sr. Anna Marie acknowledged to the floor nurse that it had been quite helpful to be informed about what to expect throughout the operating and recovery room experiences. She said that she was pleased to see a familiar face in the recovery room and that the experience had not been as lonely and frightening as she had anticipated prior to preoperative instruction.

CHAPTER 6

A WOMAN RECEIVING CHEMOTHERAPY FOR LYMPHOSARCOMA

JEAN HANYAK AND WILMA J. PHIPPS

MEDICAL HISTORY

Mrs. Mary Hart, age 61, was in good health until 5 years ago when she consulted her physician with a 5-month history of swollen nontender glands in the neck and inguinal regions. This condition was associated with pruritus and a feeling of tightness in the chest, and examination revealed hepatomegaly and splenomegaly. Mrs. Hart was subsequently hospitalized for further study, and biopsy of a cervical lymph node was diagnosed as large cell lymphosarcoma. After treatment with a course of nitrogen mustard, there was regression of lymphadenopathy and hepatosplenomegaly. A few days after discharge, however, she was readmitted with right lower-lobe pneumonia and bilateral pleural effusion. Hepatosplenomegaly recurred, and a thoracentesis was performed to relieve the pleural effusion. At this time, pleural fluid had the character of a transudate with low protein–containing lymphocytes but no malignant cells. Penicillin was used to treat the pneumonia, and because Mrs. Hart had a positive tuberculin test, prophylactic Isoniazid, 300 mg. daily, was begun.

Sixteen months after the onset of illness, Mrs. Hart was again hospitalized with recurrent pleural effusion, ascites, left arm pain, dyspnea, fatigue, and malaise. At this time, she was given a second course of nitrogen mustard and the left axilla was irradiated (1600 rad) because of probable brachial plexus compression by enlarged axillary lymph nodes. The pleural effusion and ascites were partially controlled with thiazide diuretics. She had also developed a mental depression for which antidepressants were ordered.

At the end of the second year of her illness, Mrs. Hart was readmitted because of marked increase in lymphadenopathy and hepatosplenomegaly. By this time there was neoplastic proliferation of lymphocytes into the pleura, the bone marrow, and the retroperitoneal lymph nodes. She was treated with a third course of nitrogen mustard, which was followed by the development of an anemia and leukopenia, and it was thought that this was the result of splenomegaly associated with lymphosarcoma or a combination of this factor and the effect of nitrogen mustard on bone marrow. She received two units of whole blood, which improved the hemogram. Cyclophosphamide (Cytoxan) therapy was initiated but had to be interrupted when leukopenia redeveloped. Adrenocorticosteroid therapy was then instituted with prednisone, 30 mg. daily, which was tapered off and discontinued after symptomatic improvement.

For the next 2 years Mrs. Hart received no therapy and was relatively comfortable. During this period, she attended hematology clinic at regular intervals, but at the end of this time was admitted to the hospital because of fatigue and malaise. Bilateral pleural effusion was present again, and an intravenous pyelogram showed retroperitoneal lymph node enlargement. A brief course of cyclophosphamide and prednisone was ineffective in decreasing the symptoms or the lymphocytosis (20,000). Mrs. Hart was readmitted 3 months later with weight loss, anorexia, nausea, vomiting, and night sweats—symptoms that were attributed to her primary illness, to cyclophosphamide therapy, and to mental depression. Since she had not responded to antidepressant therapy, arrangements were made for her to begin psychotherapy on an outpatient basis after discharge.

Preparations for the current admission were made by the clinic physician. In general, Mrs. Hart was progressively declining. Cytoxan was no longer effective in halting the growth of malignant cells or in providing symptomatic relief of constitutional symptoms. Therefore, it was felt that she might benefit from a course of combination chemotherapy. Mrs. Hart's chief complaints were shortness of breath and aching in the arms and legs. In addition, there was anorexia, nausea, fatigue, night sweats, and pruritus and edema of the lower extremities. She reported a weight loss of approximately 15 lb. in the last 3 months; weight on admission was 58 kg. (127.6 lb.). Her temperature then was 37.5° C. (99.5° F.). Pulse and respiration rate were normal. She had stress incontinence associated with a nonproductive cough.

PSYCHOSOCIAL BACKGROUND

Mrs. Hart, a white female, was married at the age of 25 and divorced at age 30. She and her one child, a daughter who was 2 years old at the time of the divorce, then went to live with a sister with whom she has continued to reside. Although the daughter is now married and living close by, she seldom visits and Mrs. Hart never talks about her. She does not initiate any discussion in relation to herself or to past or present experiences.

Prior to her illness, Mrs. Hart was active in her church, but since the illness has not attended church and seems to have isolated herself from the external world. She does, however, feel "gratitude and a *closeness*" toward her three sisters who take turns helping each other. The sisters keep in close touch with her and with each other; they visit regularly and telephone frequently. Mrs. Hart has never been employed and one sister, a nurse, (not the sister she lives with) supported Mrs. Hart until 1 year ago when she began to receive welfare benefits.

Mrs. Hart is aware that her disease "involves the lymph glands" and "affects the blood" and that the medication is only a "temporary relief." She has been depressed ever since she learned about "what I have." She has a good relationship with her psychotherapist who is supportive and provides an opportunity for her to "talk about my illness."

TREATMENT
Laboratory findings

Routine laboratory examination revealed several abnormal results, as follows:
Hemoglobin, 10.5 Gm./100 ml. (normal, 12 to 16).
Hematocrit, 30 vol.% (normal, 37 to 47).
White blood count, 13,500 mm.³ (normal, 4800 to 10,800).
Differential white count, normal except for the segmented neutrophils, which were 20% (normal, 50% to 70%) and the lymphocytes, which were 68% (normal, 20% to 40%).
Chest X-ray film revealed bilateral pleural effusion.
Bone marrow examination disclosed marked hyperplasia with normal elements being partially replaced by mature-appearing lymphocytes.
I.V.P. indicated that the spleen and liver were larger than previously noted; the liver now extends down to the level of the sacrum.

Medical therapy

1500 mg. sodium diet.
Isoniazid, 100 mg., t.i.d., as tuberculosis prophylaxis.
Diphenhydramine (Benadryl), 100 mg., h.s., p.r.n. for itching.
Terpin hydrate with codeine, 5 ml., p.r.n. for cough.
Trimethobenzamide (Tigan) hydrochloride suppository, 200 mg., q.4h., p.r.n. for nausea.
Restrict fluids to 2000 ml. daily.
Chemotherapy cycle on days 1 through 14:
    Nitrogen mustard, 12 mg.
    Vincristine, 1.2 mg. } I.V. on days 1 and 8.
    Prednisone, 60 mg. (20 mg. t.i.d.), on days 1 through 14.

Amobarbital, 100 mg.
Prochlorperazine dimaleate
(Compazine), 25 mg.
} orally prior to I.V. chemotherapy to reduce nausea and promote rest.

Allopurinol, 100 mg. daily, prophylactically during chemotherapy cycle to decrease uric acid excretion.

No therapy on days 15 through 28.

NURSING CARE PLAN

PROBLEM	APPROACH
Anxiety of patient and family.	Explain the nature, discomforts, and limitations of activity associated with therapeutic procedures. Listen to Mrs. Hart; encourage her to express her feelings. Assume an empathetic attitude. Promote relaxation and comfort. Remember patient's individual disorders. Encourage family to participate in Mrs. Hart's care as desired. Create a comfortable atmosphere in which family can visit.
Shortness of breath.	Use pillow if needed to support patient. Place Mrs. Hart in semi-Fowler's position; elevate head of bed. Prevent unnecessary exertion.
Edema.	Restrict oral fluids to 2000 ml. daily. Distribute fluid over 24-hour period; calculate dietary fluid; distribute remainder to make up total; reserve 200 ml. of allowed fluid to be taken at night. Elevate legs when patient is sitting in a chair. See that Mrs. Hart avoids sitting on side of bed with legs in a dependent position. Keep accurate intake and output records. Weigh every morning before breakfast. Prevent pressure and irritation of edematous areas; turn, position, and give skin care q.2h. when in bed.
Dry mouth, cracked lips.	Avoid giving irritating foods and beverages. Give frequent oral hygiene with mild cool mouthwash. Keep lips lubricated; use aromatic swabs frequently on lips and tongue. Give mouth care before and after meals.
Nausea and vomiting. Anorexia (1500 mg. sodium diet nonpalatable to patient).	Administer antiemetic—Tigan as ordered. Provide calm esthetic atmosphere at mealtime; allow extra time (eats very slowly). Talk with her and encourage her to eat (responds well to encouragement); offer small, frequent feedings.

Continued.

NURSING CARE PLAN—cont'd

PROBLEM	APPROACH
	Explain purposes of diet and importance of eating.
	Alert dietitian to food preferences.
Stress incontinence.	Offer bedpan or suggest going to bathroom frequently; provide bedside commode.
	Reassure when anxious and embarrassed.
Fatigue and weakness.	Plan nursing care to conserve patient's strength.
	Give frequent rest periods.
	Encourage ambulation activities as tolerated.
	Avoid disturbing activities and noise.
	Encourage optimal nutrition.
Bone and joint pains.	Relieve pressure of bedding by using a cradle.
	Administer hot compresses as ordered.
	Provide for joint immobilization.
Fever.	Administer cool sponges.
	Give antipyretic drugs as ordered.
	Encourage fluid intake to 2000 ml. (has been taking only about 1200 ml. daily).
	Maintain cool environmental temperature; avoid drafts.
Pruritus.	Keep patient's fingernails short.
	Use soap sparingly.
	Apply emollient lotion; pat skin dry with towel; do not rub.
Becoming less active.	Encourage personal hygiene; give her time to comb hair and clean dentures; use positive reinforcement.
Prevent side effects of cancer chemotherapy: Nausea and vomiting. Tissue slough.	Prepare for bed; give amobarbital and Compazine orally; at 10:00 P.M. have physician inject nitrogen mustard and vincristine into tubing of I.V. drip of 5% glucose in saline (run rapidly to flush drugs into vein); stay with patient; monitor I.V. site for signs of inflammation or extravasation; decrease flow rate after tubing is flushed; check patient frequently during night.

Mrs. Hart had two 14-day courses of combined therapy. Since she had experienced episodes of nausea and vomiting during previous courses of chemotherapy, she had generated a great deal of apprehension from worrying about becoming "sick" as well as from feeling that she would, and it was thought that these psychologic manifestations would enhance the development of nausea and vomiting. Much to her surprise and to the relief of the staff, however, this did not occur. Appropriate emotional support and proper physical preparation, including the administration of amobarbital and prochlorperazine dimaleate, were apparently successful in preventing this. After the first course of combined therapy, she was allowed to go home for one week, where she says she did quite well. She then returned for a second course of therapy to which she responded favorably. Her spleen became reduced in size, and there was no evidence of pleural effusion. After the second course of therapy, she was discharged to be followed in the hematology clinic weekly. Although her prognosis has been guarded, she is able to be up and about with encouragement, and she states that she feels better than she has in a long time. She will continue to see the psychiatrist on an outpatient basis.

CHAPTER 7

A WOMAN WITH CHRONIC HYPERTENSION

MARJORIE ROTT

"Oh, my head hurts so bad," moaned Mrs. Edwards as she arrived on a cart for admission at 7:45 A.M. Miss Moore, the nursing team leader, had been called by a nurse in the emergency clinic and was expecting Mrs. Edwards' transfer to the inpatient division.

Mrs. Edwards had been described as a 35-year-old black female with a 2-year history of inadequately controlled hypertension. She had been brought to the emergency clinic by her husband at 4:00 A.M., bleeding actively from the nose and complaining of severe frontal headache. On arrival her pulse was 94 and regular; blood pressure, 260/150. Meperidine hydrochloride (Demerol), 50 mg., and phenobarbital, 64 mg., were given intramuscularly at 4:30 A.M.; an ice pack was applied to the occipital area and direct lateral pressure was applied to the nares, but the nasal bleeding continued. Nasal packing was placed by an ear, nose, and throat consultant, and the epistaxis gradually slowed. Over the next 2 hours her pulse ranged from 84 to 108; blood pressure, 230/140 to 270/165. Her private physician was notified and admission to the hospital was arranged.

As Miss Moore assisted Mrs. Edwards into bed, she was beginning an assessment of her new patient's status. Mrs. Edwards' facial expression was tense; streaks of tears and serosanguineous nasal drainage were evident. Her hands moved restlessly, frequently rubbing her forehead. Answering questions quietly with short answers, she initiated comments only about intense headache pain and an unpleasant taste in her mouth. Mrs. Edwards was given an initial orientation to the room and the call light and was advised to stay in bed. Her blood pressure was 250/140 and pulse, 74, at this time. The nurse provided Mrs. Edwards with a cool facecloth and mouthwash and asked her whether she had any other requests. She explained that she would find out when medication for pain would be available and would return within 15 minutes.

As she returned to the nurses' desk, Miss Moore was mentally sorting the data she had about Mrs. Edwards, thinking, ". . . monitor vital signs, carry out drug treatment, relieve headache, bloody taste in mouth, needs sleep, . . ." as immediate goals for care. She knew that regulation of high blood pressure is essential in preventing debilitating and fatal cardiovascular complications associated with hypertension. She was on her way to review the details of the physician's plan of therapy and was wondering about her patient's background and need for readmission.

PSYCHOSOCIAL BACKGROUND

Mr. Edwards was waiting at the nurses' desk when Miss Moore returned from Mrs. Edwards' room. He asked what was being done for his wife and how she was feeling. His tense facial expression seemed to relax somewhat as Miss Moore explained that they would be checking in on Mrs. Edwards every 15 to 30 minutes for the next several hours and would be giving her medication to relieve pain and reduce her blood pressure. He wanted to see her for a moment before leaving to check with his mother who was staying with their children. Mr. Edwards left his phone number at work and indicated that he would come back to see his wife that evening. Noting his concerned expression, Miss Moore assured him of their plans for frequent observation of his wife and willingness to provide assistance. She suggested that he call later in the day for information.

Later, Miss Moore learned that Mr. Edwards is employed as a retail hardware salesman and Mrs. Edwards, as a clerk-typist. Their three children, ages 2, 6, and 9, are cared for during workdays by Mr. Edwards' mother. Both Mr. and Mrs. Edwards are high school graduates and are buying their own home. They participate actively in church and neighborhood activities.

MEDICAL HISTORY

From discussing Mrs. Edwards' care with the physician and from reading the medical records, Miss Moore gained the following additional information: Mrs. Edwards' hypertension was first diagnosed 2 years ago during her third pregnancy when she developed toxemia and her blood pressure remained elevated after parturition. She was asymptomatic, however, and did not seek medical attention until 1 year later. At that time, she presented symptoms of headache, occasional dizziness, blurred vision, a 30 lb. weight gain, and ankle edema. During this first hospitalization for hypertension she developed fever, eosinophilia, and vomiting, which subsided when methyldopa (Aldomet) was discontinued. She was discharged on a combination of guanethidine sulfate (Ismelin) and Dyazide.

Four months later readmission was necessary because of poor blood pressure control, the recurrence of intermittent blurred vision, and pedal edema. She had continued to work, however, until headaches increased in severity and increasing doses of furosemide (Lasix) failed to prove effective in relieving her symptoms. At discharge her blood pressure was 210/135 to 190/120 on a combination of guanethidine, Dyazide, and phenoxybenzamine hydrochloride (Dibenzyline).

When she was seen in the physician's office prior to this third and present admission, blood pressure control remained poor, ranging from 230/120 to 250/130. Mrs. Edwards' only symptom, however, was occasional headache. On this admission, physical examination and evaluation revealed the following:

Slightly obese, 35-year-old black female.

Epistaxis—posterior nasal pack in place, slight oozing.

Hypertensive since toxemia 2 years ago.

BP (right arm)—sitting, 240/128; standing, 250/130.

No postural hypotension, as would be expected with Dibenzyline and guanethidine.

No scleral icterus or periorbital edema; no petechiae.

Occasional leg edema.

No venous neck distention.

Prominent systolic thrust; ECG—left ventricular hypertrophy.

No rhonchi, no rales.

Sensorium clear; severe frontal headache.

No allergies; smokes ½ pack of cigarettes daily.

TREATMENT
Medical therapy

The immediate goal in medical therapy was to lower Mrs. Edwards' blood pressure by means of intramuscular reserpine and morphine. Oral antihypertensive and diuretic medications were instituted concurrently, working toward establishing the maintenance doses needed for long-range blood pressure regulation. This goal of therapy was aimed toward control of the chronic hypertension and prevention of further complications. Treatment of the present epistaxis was underway; supervision by the ear, nose, and throat consultant was continued.

The following are the physician's orders for the medical care of Mrs. Edwards:

April 9
8:30 A.M.   *Diagnosis.* Chronic hypertension, uncontrolled epistaxis secondary to hypertension.

Morphine sulfate, 10 mg., I.M., now, and q.3h. p.r.n. for pain or agitation.

	Reserpine (Serpasil), 1 mg., I.M., now.
	BP, q.1h.; P and T, q.4h.
10:00 A.M.	Fair condition.
	Regular diet with no added salt.
	Bed rest with head elevated.
	Intake and output.

Lab tests now and in morning: hemoglobin, hematocrit, fasting blood
   sugar, BUN, Na, K, Cl, CO_2.

Chest X-ray.

ECG.

Urinalysis.

Report if BP less than 110 diastolic.

Medication:

    Guanethidine sulfate, 100 mg., p.o., q.d.

    Phenoxybenzamine HCl, 40 mg., p.o., q.d.

    Dyazide, 2 capsules, p.o., q.d.

    Maalox, 30 ml., p.o., q.i.d., 1 hour p. c., and h.s.

    Secobarbital, 100 mg., p.o., h.s., p.r.n.

    Milk of magnesia, 30 ml., p.o., h.s., p.r.n.

    Darvon, 65 mg., p.o., q.4h., p.r.n.

4:00 P.M.   Reserpine, 1 mg., I.M., now.

    Pentazocine, 30 mg., I.M., q.4h., p.r.n. for pain.

April 10

12:30 A.M.   Repeat reserpine, 1 mg., I.M., now.

10:00 A.M.   Reserpine, 1 mg., I.M., now.

2:00 P.M.   BP, q.2h. × 4; if stable, q.4h.

    Ear, nose, and throat consultant to see in morning.

April 11

11:00 A.M.   Reserpine, 1 mg., I.M., now.

    Increase guanethidine sulfate to 125 mg. p.o., q.d.

    Morphine, 6 mg., I.M., now and q.3h. p.r.n.

    BP q.i.d.

April 12

9:00 A.M.   Increase guanethidine sulfate to 150 mg., p.o., q.d.

    Up in room slowly, as tolerated.

PROGRESSIVE NURSING INTERVENTIONS

Miss Moore located Miss Hawkins, the nurse on their patient care team who would be assigned to Mrs. Edwards, and shared the preliminary information with her. They discussed Mrs. Edwards' immediate needs for close observation and relief of discomfort and formulated a beginning plan of care. With plans to revise the care plan as Mrs. Edwards' condition changed and/or more data was available, Miss Moore noted their ideas in the Kardex to be available for other staff members. The initial nursing care plan appears on p. 36.

INITIAL NURSING CARE PLAN
April 9, Mrs. J. Edwards

DATA/OBSERVATIONS	OBJECTIVES	NURSING ACTIONS
Diagnosis. Hypertension unregulated.	Monitor condition. Promote medical therapy.	Take BP and P. q.½-1h. Notify doctor if diastolic BP rises in 3 consecutive readings or falls below 110. Administer medications and nursing care at times of vital signs to minimize interrupting rest. Avoid noise, haste, and bright lights.
Headache pain.	Minimize discomfort.	Assess need for p.r.n. pain medication q.2-3h.; assess verbal requests, tenseness, and restlessness.
Bloody oozing from nose.	Reduce bleeding.	Change ice pack and cool facecloth at bedside q.2-3h. and p.r.n.
Nausea.	Minimize nausea.	Resupply mouthwash and mouthcare equipment at bedside p.r.n. Try liquid diet, iced fluids, and frequent mouth care; remind to expectorate bloody postnasal drainage.
Fatigue and loss of sleep.	Provide for rest and quiet.	Combine nursing care activities to minimize interruptions. Identify other actions for comfort—dim light, door closed, positioned head up.

A graphic sheet was posted at the nurses' station for recording Mrs. Edwards' vital signs in a place accessible to all staff monitoring her condition. Within 72 hours of intensive medical management and nursing care, Mrs. Edwards' physical condition stabilized. Her blood pressure stayed within an acceptable range, 190/90 to 160/115, her nasal bleeding had stopped and the packing was removed, and she was generally fairly comfortable.

While getting up out of bed slowly and for short intervals, or while walking in her room unaided, she experienced only occasional headaches and transient dizziness. Mrs. Edwards' kidney function test results were reported within the lower limits of normal and her blood values were within normal ranges. She talked frequently about her family and of the many things she wanted to be doing at home. She expressed both satisfaction with feeling so much better and eagerness to go home and get back to the "normal routines." She did not mention previous hospitalizations or symptoms, but occasionally asked the nurse about the blood pressure reading as it was being taken.

The physician felt that Mrs. Edwards' chronic hypertension could be controlled with medication and without drastic changes in life style. Continued evaluation and health supervision, along with adjustments in drug therapy, could minimize hypertensive complications and progression of cardiovascular damage.

As Mrs. Edwards' physical condition improved, the nursing staff reevaluated their goals and plan of nursing care. It was agreed that increasing emphasis needed to be placed on longer range goals for her care outside the hospital. Information already available included Mrs. Edwards' history of three admissions within 9 months because of symptoms of uncontrolled hypertension. Because of the chronic nature of the disease and the necessity for continued therapy, the outcome for Mrs. Edwards rested, to a great degree, on her adherence to the prescribed medical regimen. The goal of teaching responsibility for her own well-being was clearly identified. However, the questions surrounding why this had not previously been achieved remained unanswered.

To teach self-care, the staff first identified their need to know more about Mrs. Edwards. As the nursing team discussed their ideas, they found they did have some data and observations of her behavior from which to start planning their further data collection and "teaching plans." They presented the significant data they already had about this individual: her many family, work, and community responsibilities and activities; her seeking medical attention for only severe symptoms; the lack of conversation about treatment and past problems, and only an occasional expression of interest in her condition. A care plan to be followed with the patient was written out to summarize the nursing staff's thoughts and to identify areas needing further evaluation.

PROGRESSIVE NURSING CARE PLAN
April 12, Mrs. J. Edwards

DATA	OBJECTIVES	NURSING ACTIONS
Diagnosis. Uncontrolled hypertension. Third admission in 9 months with complications. Seeks medical attention when symptoms interfere with functioning. Probably irregular self-administration of medications. "Concerned about care of family, job." "Likes to be active" and to get work done.	Identify perception of illness.	Identify Mrs. Edwards' understanding of: Effects of disease. Natural course of disease without treatment. Relation of her symptoms—headache, nosebleed, pedal edema, emesis, fatigue—to underlying disease. Possibility of fear of disease.
Occasionally asks about BP reading.	Identify self-care learning needs. Plan teaching-learning opportunities. Offer information in "usable manner." Identify possible helpful reinforcement.	Identify Mrs. Edwards' readiness and personal goals for learning. Set mutually acceptable times for planned discussions. Relate medical schedule to work and home activities; use American Heart Association booklets as a source of specific information on diet, home activities, etc. Explore visits by the nurse from the Visiting Nurses' Association after discharge.
Husband concerned about wife's progress.	Identify priority information to be taught. Have him sit in on teaching sessions when possible.	Teach the following: Chronicity of disease—patient's role in control. Control is possible with drug therapy. Side effects of medications:

PROGRESSIVE NURSING CARE PLAN—cont'd
April 12, Mrs. J. Edwards

DATA	OBJECTIVES	NURSING ACTIONS
		Guanethidine—postural hypotension, diarrhea, nausea. Phenoxybenzamine—postural hypotension. Dyazide—dizziness. Effects of overweight, worry, and smoking on BP. How to minimize episodes of postural hypotension: Allow extra time to rise from lying to standing position. Sit up slowly in bed. Dangle feet over side of bed for a few minutes. Stand up slowly. If dizzy or faint, sit down and put head between knees. Keep record of episodes and report them to doctor. Medication dosage may have to be adjusted if episodes are frequent. Carry a card or wear a Medic-Alert bracelet, which should give: Name, address, phone number, name and address of physicians, medications being taken and their dosage.

Continued.

PROGRESSIVE NURSING CARE PLAN—cont'd
April 12, Mrs. J. Edwards

DATA	OBJECTIVES	NURSING ACTIONS
		Family and employer should know what medications can cause dizziness or fainting; they should know what to do if this occurs.

With these potential goals for nursing intervention written out, a guide for deliberate action was available to all personnel interacting with Mrs. Edwards. Alternative courses of action were made available as a stimulus to the staff in the information gathering and analysis. Miss Moore, the team leader, was designated to coordinate their findings.

CHAPTER 8

A MAN WITH A
POSSIBLE MYOCARDIAL INFARCTION

FRANCES R. BROWN

MEDICAL HISTORY

Mr. Charles was admitted to the coronary care unit (CCU) with intermittent, sharp precordial pain and "palpitations." He has a history of cardiovascular disease—one myocardial infarction, cardiomegaly, and hypertension. He also has a family history of arteriosclerotic heart disease. Mr. Charles smokes two packs of cigarettes a day and drinks heavily.

While in the hospital, Mr. Charles experienced several episodes of precordial pain that were precipitated by activity or emotional distress. He responded negatively to medical therapy and nursing care in the CCU and was transferred 6 days after admission to a general medical-surgical unit with a diagnosis of coronary artery disease.

PSYCHOSOCIAL BACKGROUND

Mr. Charles is a gray-haired, muscular man who lives in his own home with his wife. Their only child, a daughter, died of cancer a year ago, leaving a husband and three children. Mr. Charles cried several times when discussing the daughter and stated that his grandchildren were growing up to be rude and "spoiled." He works at a drill company where he handles heavy equipment, but plans to retire in 6 months, after his sixty-fifth birthday. Several times he stated that he has problems that are "more pressing" than his hospitalization, and he remained stoic about his health. In addition, Mr. Charles disregarded limitations placed on his activity by the physician.

TREATMENT
Medical therapy

Elastic stockings, footboard, leg exercises.
Bed rest at first and then activity as tolerated.

Medications
    Dioctyl sodium succinate (Colace), 100 mg., t.i.d.
    Isosorbide dinitrate (Isodril), 5 mg., q.i.d.
    Chlordiazepoxide (Librium), 10 mg., t.i.d.
    Pentazocine (Talwin), 50 mg., or Darvon, 65 mg., q.4h., p.r.n. for pain.
    Secobarbital (Seconal), 100 mg., h.s., p.r.n.

Laboratory findings

ECG
    Sinus rhythm with intermittent left bundle branch block and frequent
        premature ventricular contractions.
Blood
    Glucose, 110 to 125 mg./100 ml. (normal, 65 to 110).
    Serum glutamic oxaloacetic transaminase, 16 to 25 units over 5-day period
        (normal, 9 to 25 units).
    Lactic dehydrogenase, 62 to 70 units over 5-day period (normal, 40 to 100
        units).
    Erythrocytes, 4.5 million/mm.[3] (normal, 4.6 to 6.2).
    Hematocrit, 45 vol.% (normal, 40 to 54).

NURSING INTERVENTION: OBJECTIVES AND RATIONALE FOR NURSING ACTION

To reduce fear by acquainting Mr. Charles with the environment. Coronary
care units can be frightening to patients because of their fear of the unknown
and the presence of strange equipment. The nurse who admitted Mr. Charles introduced herself and explained the cardiac monitor in simple terms as she attached it. She gave him time to ask questions and, after taking his vital signs,
told him generally what he could expect during his stay in the unit. As Mr.
Charles described his pain, the nurse observed him for signs of distress and then
elicited a brief history of his illness. She also determined that he was allergic
to penicillin.

To reduce the workload of his heart. Mr. Charles' ECG showed evidence of
ischemia to the cardiac conducting system (intermittent left bundle branch
block) and myocardial irritability (premature ventricular contractions). Precordial pain upon exertion (angina pectoris) also indicated that Mr. Charles'
coronary circulation was impaired. Thus, modified bed rest was ordered.

Modified bed rest (allowing a patient to feed himself and use a bedside commode) and alternating periods of activity with rest periods reduces the body's
requirement for oxygen, thus reducing the workload of the heart. When oxygen

demands are decreased, a damaged heart often can pump sufficient blood to meet body needs. When the blood supply to the myocardium is adequate, anginal pain subsides. Mr. Charles' low hematocrit value may have been a factor contributing to his pain because there were fewer erythrocytes to carry oxygen. His serum enzyme (SGOT and LDH) values and ECG showed no evidence of a recent myocardial infarction.

To prevent thromboembolic complications in the lower extremities. Bed rest is a predisposing factor in the development of peripheral vascular problems because of inactive muscles and pooling of blood. A footboard, active and passive exercises, and elastic stockings were used to enhance venous return to the heart by compressing the veins and to maintain muscle tone.

To encourage Mr. Charles to verbalize his fears and concerns. Mr. Charles had family and retirement problems in addition to cardiac disease, and the medical and nursing staff described him as being belligerent. At this time, he was receiving isosorbide dinitrate, which gave him severe headaches. As the dosage of isosorbide dinitrate was decreased, the headaches became less severe and his behavior became more positive. The nurses provided opportunities for him to verbalize his feelings and often served as a "sounding board." They collaborated with physicians and with a Medicare worker in an effort to meet this patient's needs.

To observe general guidelines for care of a patient with a myocardial infarction who is being monitored electronically.

Vital signs
   Take apical pulse for a full minute.
   When patient's temperature is 38° C. (100° F.) or above, take rectal temperature.
      Position patient on side.
      Insert rectal thermometer gently after lubricating it well.
   Monitor vital signs (especially pulse) before, during, and after activity.
Intravenous fluids
   When I.V. tubing is present, change dressing daily, cleanse area with antiseptic, and apply Bacitracin ointment.
   Apply moist heat to area when inflammation is present.
   Avoid disconnecting I.V. tubing unless essential for monitoring central venous pressure or for a specific treatment.
Electrical safety
   Use only equipment that has been properly grounded (3-prong plug).
   Avoid using 3-prong plug adaptors.
   If an extra grounding cable must be used, attach it only to an unpainted

water pipe or to a specific copper grounding pipe. Oxygen outlets, electrical outlets, patients' beds, and painted radiators are unacceptable "grounds."

Always disconnect patient cable from ECG machine while leads are being placed on patient who is also attached to a cardiac monitor. Just before ECG is to be recorded, disconnect patient cable from monitor and then attach patient cable to ECG machine.

Cardiac monitor

Change electrodes at least every 24 hours in most situations.

Remove electrodes.

Clean and dry skin.

Apply fresh paste and electrodes.

Be sure that alarm systems are turned on.

External pacemaker

Cover any exposed wires.

Support patient's arm and shoulder to prevent dislodging of pacing catheter.

Psychologic considerations

Adapt care to patient's needs.

Maintain subdued-to-normal lighting.

Provide information needed to help patient and family adjust to unit.

Provide opportunity for patient and family to express their feelings.

Mr. Charles was discharged from the hospital 2 weeks after admission. Although family problems were still present, he had received some help from the staff who attempted to assist him in solving them. Mr. Charles could not give up smoking, which was not surprising for a man of his age who had smoked for "50 years." He was, however, able to moderate his smoking and had decreased the number of cigarettes from two packs to less than one pack per day. He was discharged on a 1500-calorie diet with pentaerythritol tetranitrate (Peritrate) tablets, one to be taken on arising and one 12 hours later.

CHAPTER 9

AN ELDERLY WOMAN WHO REQUIRED PERMANENT PACEMAKER THERAPY

SANDRA S. SHUMWAY

MEDICAL HISTORY

Mrs. Lowell is an 85-year-old woman who has been attending the outpatient clinic for many years. Her initial medical diagnoses included arteriosclerotic cardiovascular disease, myocardial hypertrophy, episodes of congestive heart failure (CHF), and chronic ankle edema. She was hospitalized 3 years ago after the development of pulmonary edema secondary to a myocardial infarction. A left bundle branch block (LBBB) was observed by ECG in the course of her hospitalization. She was discharged in 2 weeks after a smooth recovery. Six weeks later she returned to the outpatient clinic for her first visit. While in the clinic she suffered a cardiac arrest secondary to ventricular fibrillation. She was resuscitated promptly, but developed a complete heart block (CHB) with an idioventricular rate of 45 beats per minute. The block did not subside and therefore a permanent transvenous pacemaker was eventually inserted. The pacemaker was of the fixed-rate type and was set to stimulate the myocardium at 72 beats per minute. The pacemaker battery was implanted, under local anesthesia, between the fascia of the pectoralis major muscle and the subcutaneous tissue of the left chest wall just superior to the breast in the anterior axillary line. The transvenous catheter electrode was tunneled beneath the subcutaneous tissue and inserted into the left external jugular vein, where it coursed via the subclavian and innominate veins to the superior vena cava and right atrium and then to the right ventricle where the catheter tip was wedged in the muscular bands.

Several complications ensued in the postoperative period. The original electrode stimulated the phrenic nerve and Mrs. Lowell experienced diaphragmatic spasm over a long period of time. After the pacemaker electrode was replaced, she expressed fear of being hurt by the "electricity" in the pacemaker and used a stiff gait while ambulating. In addition, her neck incision developed a slight serous drainage and seemed to cause quite a bit of pain. Mrs. Lowell wondered whether she would ever be able to manage at home, and she appeared slightly depressed during part of her convalescence.

PSYCHOSOCIAL BACKGROUND

Mrs. Lowell is an elderly woman who usually exhibits boundless energy in her daily activities. She possesses a quiet enthusiasm for living that is contagious. She lives in a small apartment in a large urban area where she has lived for most of her adult life. She is an active member of the Methodist church. Her religious faith is strong and is a source of strength for her in periods of stress. When she became eligible for social security benefits, she began doing volunteer work for many organizations in the community. Her only remaining family are two sisters who live in the East. She has numerous friends whom she feels free to call upon for support.

Mrs. Lowell attends the outpatient clinics regularly. In the first year of her visits to the clinic, she developed a digitalis toxicity in the course of the therapy she was receiving for an episode of congestive heart failure. She subsequently stopped taking digitalis preparations because she feared a repetition of the symptoms related to the toxicity and because she had promised herself that if she became well after the toxicity episode she would never take "those pills" again. Her CHF has been controlled effectively with a sodium-restricted diet and a diuretic. The patient places a great deal of faith in home remedies. She learned this in her youth, since her mother treated all her illnesses with "herbs from the woods." Mrs. Lowell reported that she took the prescribed drugs (including a preparation of digitalis) for a "few days" after her discharge from the hospital after the myocardial infarction. Once the pacemaker had been inserted, she expressed the feeling that her current problems had been caused by taking too much digitalis. Furthermore, she could not recall giving permission for the pacemaker therapy and did not feel she needed it.

TREATMENT
Medical therapy

The patient was discharged with instructions to take hydrochlorothiazide (HydroDiuril), 50 mg., once a day. She was encouraged to eat foods high in potassium each day and to avoid added salt in her diet. In addition, she was urged to ambulate to the point of tiring.

Laboratory findings

Prior to her discharge Mrs. Lowell's laboratory data revealed the following: Blood urea nitrogen, 13 mg./100 ml. (normal range, 10 to 15).

Sodium, 135 mEq./L. (normal, 137 to 143).

Potassium, 3.7 mEq./L. (normal, 4 to 5).

Chloride, 98 mEq./L. (normal, 98 to 103).

Serum glutamic oxaloacetic transaminase, 23 units (normal, less than 40).

Hemoglobin, 12 Gm./100 ml. (normal, 12 to 16).

Hematocrit, 38 vol.% (normal, 36 to 47).

Total leukocytes, 7650 (normal, 5000 to 10,000).

NURSING INTERVENTION

The objectives that follow were developed for the convalescent stage of Mrs. Lowell's illness—the period of time just prior to discharge and during the initial months at home. These objectives for intervention are selective in that they focus upon only two broad areas of concern. The first area deals with facilitating Mrs. Lowell's initial return home to live as independently as possible and with decreasing fear of the pacemaker. The second is related to the assessment of her cardiovascular status by the nurse and to the teaching that was required to assist Mrs. Lowell in understanding her therapy as she learned how to evaluate her own cardiac status. Objectives for other aspects of care that might be derived from a review of the history are not included.

Two objectives for nursing intervention

1. To provide the support Mrs. Lowell requires to assist her in returning to live and manage her own life needs with decreasing fear and awareness of the pacemaker.

Discussion. The health history reveals that Mrs. Lowell is an elderly person. She may, therefore, possess diminished physical and emotional resources to draw upon in coping with abrupt changes. This is an especially important factor as she did not recall giving permission for the therapy. She had experienced an acute illness and was frightened by the prescribed therapy (the pacemaker). Her fear may also have been reinforced by her experience with the discomfort of the diaphragmatic stimulation. This episode of stimulation may have confirmed her feeling that the pacemaker stimuli might harm her.

Her history also indicates that she walks in a stiff manner. This may be evidence of her fear that the pacemaker might harm her, or of her concern about the sensation experienced by movement of the pacemaker battery pack as the muscles of her chest wall contract, or of her fear of falling after spending a period of limited activity, a common concern in the older person.[11]

Her laboratory findings reveal normal values, with the exception of the slightly low serum potassium (K^+) level. The serum K^+ does, however, fall within a low normal level. Despite this fact, subsequent K+ levels should be reviewed. In addition, since serum K+ is not an accurate indication of deficiency of K+, consideration must also be given to other clinical evidence of K+ loss, such as symptoms associated with the nerve conduction disturbances and symptoms associated with disturbances in the function of cardiac and skeletal muscle.[9] Finally, K+ loss may be associated with the administration of certain diuretics. Mrs. Lowell will need help in understanding the need to follow through in this particular aspect of her dietary recommendations.

Specific nursing intervention

a. Develop with Mrs. Lowell and the nursing staff a plan that will help Mrs. Lowell to increase her activities in the hospital and at home in a progressive manner. While she is increasing her activity level, observe her ability to handle increasing physical exertion by monitoring her cardiovascular status through assessment of blood pressure (observe for hypotension and syncope) and pulse (observe for arrhythmias and bradycardia or tachycardia). Other visible signs of physiologic functioning that should be noted are color of skin (marked pallor), mentation (confusion, dizziness, excess arousal), coordination of gait (staggering), an excess fatigue or angina[6] as she increases her participation in activities of daily living (ADL). Scan her laboratory findings regularly to detect other indicators that might also account for signs of muscular dysfunction, such as fatigue, staggering, and cardiac arrhythmias (low serum K+).

b. Suggest a leave of absence from the hospital for increasing periods of time to help Mrs. Lowell achieve confidence in her ability to manage independently. Work closely with her in planning the appropriate time for this. Encourage her to contact friends that could help her. Call the Visiting Nurses' Association concerning follow-up after discharge. Invite a visiting nurse to meet with the patient and staff in the hospital. Work with the visiting nurse and with Mrs. Lowell to develop plans for management of responsibilities at home. Consider using a homemaker to assist her with housekeeping activities after discharge. This might be especially appropriate in view of her age and her initial difficulty in ambulating. Develop an awareness of the need for the patient to receive praise as she progresses slowly toward independence.

c. Provide opportunities for Mrs. Lowell to ask questions about her pacemaker. Each member of the staff will need to be informed about answers to the questions she is likely to ask and about which her family and friends will be most concerned. For example, Mrs. Lowell needs to know that repositioning of the electrode will stop the muscular spasms and that the pacemaker stimuli are not strong enough to harm her. If she expresses an interest, a schematic picture can be drawn to show the placement of the pacemaker battery and the electrode. She may need reassurance that pacemakers have been used in many other people and that this is not an uncommon therapy. She will also need to know that while the lump in her chest will be noticeable, in time she will not be as aware of the pacemaker as she is now.

d. If Mrs. Lowell seems uncomfortable as she walks around, it may be caused by the dragging sensation or heavy feeling that some patients experience from the pull of the weight of the pacemaker battery on the tissue of the chest wall. Some patients have been relieved of this sensation by using a soft brassiere that supports the weight of the pacemaker while supporting the breast tissue. The brassiere should not be worn until the incision line has healed, however, and the bra should be changed frequently during hot weather to avoid any rubbing over the incision line even though it is healed. The patient may need the nurses' support as well as guidance in using this approach, as some elderly women may have discontinued the use of a brassiere.

2. *To make accurate nursing assessments of Mrs. Lowell's cardiovascular status over time and to help her learn how to evaluate her own cardiac status.*

Discussion. The health history reveals that Mrs. Lowell had a myocardial infarction and subsequent complete heart block (CHB) with a rate of 45 beats per minute. Pacemaker therapy was instituted initially because CHB with a myocardial infarction is reported by some to be associated with a higher mortality than acute myocardial infarction alone. Long-term pacemaker therapy is felt to be useful in preventing CHF secondary to a slow rate.[4]

Mrs. Lowell is also receiving 50 mg. of hydrochlorothiazide each day to treat her CHF. In view of her past history regarding drugs, she will need observation concerning the medication regime.

Although the etiology of third-degree block is reported to be poorly understood,[10] the atrioventricular block of the older person may result from degeneration and fibrosis in the area of the valvular rings of the heart.[2] Although heart block associated with acute myocardial infarction is frequently a transient phenomenon,[3] Mrs. Lowell's heart block persisted, and it was necessary to implant a permanent pacemaker. In view of her age and the chronic nature of her cardiac problem, it might be anticipated that Mrs. Lowell will require the pacemaker for as long as she lives.

The pacemaker used to treat Mrs. Lowell was of the fixed-rate type. (Descriptions of pacemaker equipment, function, and methods of implantation are reported elsewhere.[5,7]) The rate of this pacemaker should be consistent over time. The health history notes that Mrs. Lowell had a heart rate of 72 beats per minute on discharge. A change in rate of 5 to 10 beats per minute may be indicative of pacemaker failure.[1] Mrs. Lowell will need to be prepared for the fact that the pacemaker battery pack may require changing within 18 to 30 months, or whenever signs of altered function are noted. The health history also reveals that Mrs. Lowell felt depressed during her convalescence. As previously noted, she did not remember giving permission for the pacemaker implant. Her depression may be indicative of feelings associated with lack of control over her current situation.

Specific nursing intervention

a. Develop a method for making systematic assessments of cardiovascular status and pacemaker function. Each time Mrs. Lowell is observed, record evidence of stability in cardiovascular status; take the apical pulse, blood pressure, respiration, and weight; and compare them with the last recording. Observe for pulse rate increase over time or a sudden change in rate that might indicate beginning failure of the pacemaker batteries. Observe and record signs of CHF that might be secondary to pacemaker failure. These signs include shortness of breath, cough, insomnia, anorexia, paroxysmal nocturnal dyspnea, fatigue, dependent edema, and weight increase (these last two are late signs[8]). Share findings in writing and verbally with Mrs. Lowell's physician and work with him in developing future plans. Share findings and plans with the visiting nurse if she is involved.

b. Help Mrs. Lowell to understand the reason for her pacemaker and to evaluate her own cardiac status over time. In view of Mrs. Lowell's initial fear about the pacemaker and her possible feelings concerning lack of control over her current health situation, it might be advisable to start teaching her how to take her own pulse. The nursing staff could talk with her about her pulse when they are checking it. The nurses' aide, the physician, and others on the health team should be aware of this plan, but specific members of the staff should work closely with Mrs. Lowell. Doing so will facilitate evaluation of her progress. In addition, this relationship will provide the support Mrs. Lowell needs and give her opportunities to ask questions. The goal is to work toward having Mrs. Lowell take her pulse once daily and to record it to bring to her physician. She should also understand the need to check her pulse if she does not feel well or if she has a dizzy spell. This information will help the physician determine whether there is a pacemaker malfunction.

When the patient seems to be comfortable while checking her own pulse, and when she expresses interest in other aspects of the therapy (for example, by raising questions), help her to understand the meaning of her heart rate and the need to contact her physician if the heart rate should vary by 5 to 10 beats per minute. In time, she should learn to report other evidence of alterations in cardiovascular status such as unusual fatigue, edema and weight gain, nocturia, anorexia, dizzy spells, or syncope. Although infection in the operative area is not common, Mrs. Lowell will need to learn the signs of infection. A matter-of-fact approach helps the patient feel more comfortable about checking his own status.

c. Mrs. Lowell should also be prepared for the fact that she will require a periodic replacement of the battery pack. Since many persons worry about this, the nurse will need to spend time helping Mrs. Lowell to talk about the anticipated surgery. Although local anesthesia is used, patients are often frightened by the procedure and require a good deal of support. If Mrs. Lowell is upset, one of the nurses who has been working with her should accompany her to the operating room.

d. Work with Mrs. Lowell to help her understand the purpose of the hydrochlorothiazide therapy. Help her to develop a specific regimen for taking the drug each day and for including in her daily diet foods high in potassium (for example orange juice, raisins, bananas) so as to avoid hypokalemia associated with diuretic therapy. One way to help her remember to take her medication each day would be for her to associate taking it with an important event such as when she checks her pulse, or at mealtimes.

Helping Mrs. Lowell increase her awareness of the need for drug therapy is of crucial importance. She has a history of failure to take drugs for reasons that are understandable. However, she might continue to avoid drug therapy if she does not see the reason for it and, of more importance perhaps, if she feels the need to control her therapy in some way, since she is unable to remove the pacemaker.

Review current blood chemistries to detect changes indicative of electrolyte imbalance. Also evaluate clinical signs of hypokalemia as noted previously.

RESULTS OF NURSING INTERVENTION

Mrs. Lowell was able to learn to take her pulse, but only after 12 months had passed following the pacemaker implant. She was so frightened of the pacemaker therapy that she needed to deny its existence for this period of time. Once she felt comfortable with the therapy, she quickly learned to take her own pulse and to evaluate her cardiac status.

Close collaboration between professionals involved in her care facilitated an understanding of the various steps in her progress toward independence. It also facilitated early detection of signs of pacemaker malfunction and development of plans to meet her ever-changing needs. The systematic assessment of her cardiovascular status over a period of time helped to increase understanding of the insidious changes in pulse rate and behavior that sometimes signal pacemaker failure.

Finally, the staff's close work with Mrs. Lowell provided her with the opportunity to find answers to questions that puzzled her and to find the support needed by an elderly woman receiving therapy that frightened her and her family and friends.

REFERENCES

1. Bluestone, R., Harris, A., and Davis, G.: Aftercare of artificially paced patients, Brit. Med. J. 1:1589-1594, June 1965.
2. Carelton, R. A., Sessions, R. W., and Graettinger, J. S.: Cardiac pacemaker: clinical and physiological studies, Med. Clin. N. Amer. 50:325-1110, Jan. 1966.
3. Carlson, R. G., and others: Results of cardiac surgery in 273 older patients, Geriatrics 22: 173-183, Oct. 1967.
4. Friedberg, L. K., Cohen, H., and Donosa, E.: Advanced heart block as a complication of acute myocardial infarction: role of pacemaker therapy, Progr. Cardiovas. Dis. 10:466-481, March 1968.
5. Germain, C. J., and Hanley, Sr. M. P.: Metronome for a music teacher, Amer. J. Nurs. 68:498-503, March 1968.
6. Hellerstein, H. K., and Hornstein, T. R.: Assessing and preparing the patient for return to a meaningful, productive life, J. Rehab. 32:48-52, March-April 1966.
7. Hunn, V. K.: Cadiac pacemakers, Amer. J. Nurs. 69:749-754, April 1969.
8. Hurst, J. W., and Logue, R. B.: The heart, arteries and veins, New York, 1970, McGraw-Hill Book Co.
9. MacBryde, C. M. (editor): Signs and symptoms, ed. 4, Philadelphia, 1964, J. B. Lippincott Co.
10. Stillman, M. T.: Transvenous pacing of the heart, Minn. Med. 51:127-136, Jan. 1968.
11. Ujhely, G. B.: Determinants of the nurse patient relationship, New York, 1968, Springer Publishing Co., Inc.

CHAPTER 10

CONGESTIVE HEART FAILURE AND PULMONARY EDEMA IN AN ELDERLY MAN

ARDITH SUDDUTH

MEDICAL HISTORY

Mr. Peter Hunt, a married 81-year-old white male, was admitted late in the afternoon to a semiprivate room with the diagnosis of congestive heart failure with pulmonary edema. His chief complaint on admission was severe shortness of breath on exertion and inability to sleep for the past three nights. Shortly after his admission and during the evening, the following information was collected from Mr. Hunt, his chart, and his physician to facilitate planning his nursing care:

Respiratory status

Respirations—28 to 32/min. with effort; using shoulder and neck muscles to facilitate breathing.

Two-year history of two-pillow orthopnea.

Position of comfort—sitting at 45-degree angle.

Wet, diffuse rales heard halfway up the anterior and posterior thorax.

O_2 running at 2 L./min.

Dyspnea with talking; respiratory effort interrupts talking.

No cough.

Never smoked.

Temperature

37.5° C. (99.5° F.) orally.

Circulatory status

BP—130/180; left brachial artery at 45-degree angle while he is lying in bed.

Pulse—96 for left radial, slightly irregular and weak; 105 for apical, slightly irregular and difficult to hear; no pulses palpable below femorals.

Taking the following *medications* at home:
>   Nitroglycerin, 1 or 2 tablets q.d. for 10 years; required for exertion such as walking up a flight of stairs or being "emotionally upset."
>   Digoxin, 0.25 mg. q.d. for 2 years.
>   Ethacrynic acid (Edecrin), 50 mg. q.d. for 1 week.
>   KCl solution, q.d. for 1 week.

Feet and legs slightly edematous.
Hepatomegaly.
Ascites.

Nutritional status
Weight—70.3 kg. (154.6 lb.) on admission at 4:00 P.M. (standing weight in own pajamas).
Height—172.5 cm. (5 feet, 6½ inches).
Appetite "poor" for several weeks.
No added salt diet at home for 2 years; uses salt substitute.
Likes warm milk at h.s. and on cereal at breakfast.
Occasionally drinks alcohol socially.
Never drinks ice water or eats ice cream because of angina pain.
Sanka coffee, hot tea.
Edentulous; full upper and lower dentures; takes out only at night to soak in cleansing solution brought to hospital with him.
No allergies to drugs or foods.

Skin
Pale and clammy.
Intact, clean.
Dry and taut over feet and lower legs.
Hair loss on legs.
Thin, balding pattern of scalp.
Well-groomed, immaculately kept man.
Showers daily at home.
Shaves daily in morning with electric razor.

Sensory
Wears glasses only for reading.
Hears speaking voice across room (approximately 12 to 18 feet).

Motor
Walks unassisted.
Functional range of motion in all joints.
"I've always been tired."
Prior to onset of acute illness 1 week ago, became tired and had some angina pain while walking the one block from his parking garage to his office.

Rest and comfort status

Sleeps 12:00 midnight or 1:00 A.M. to 10:00-11:00 A.M. at home.

Two pillows, electric blanket.

Warm milk at 11:00 P.M.-12:00 midnight each night.

Has own room at home.

Elimination

Difficulty starting urinary stream; must stand to void.

Daily BM after 11:00 A.M.-12:00 noon meal.

Occasionally takes milk of magnesia at night.

PSYCHOSOCIAL BACKGROUND

Social status

81-year-old white male.

Continues to operate his own business from his home and downtown office.

Goes to office two to three times a week.

Drives to office in own automobile equipped with power steering, power brakes, and automatic transmission.

Wife has been an invalid for 10 years.

Practical nurse/housekeeper in home 24 hours per day.

No children.

Many friends in city; several phone calls from friends first hours of his admission.

Study and bedroom on second floor of home.

Six months ago had power elevator chair installed for himself and his wife to facilitate going up and down stairs.

Physician describes his social life as "active."

Mental status

Alert and oriented.

Describes by name medications he has been taking and their action.

Describes his angina pectoris and types of exertion giving pain.

Describes current illness as "heart weakness."

Three years of college education.

Reads newspaper daily.

Attention span short.

Talks about himself with comfort and ease.

Emotional status

Concern over continuing shortness of breath and difficulty breathing.

Difficulty resting.

Wide-eyed, "apprehensive" look on face upon admission.

TREATMENT
Diagnostic tests
ECG—showed a rapid heart rate (105) with occasional premature ventricular beats, some abberant supraventricular premature beats, and left
bundle branch block.
Chest X-ray—(taken on his way to division) showed large bilateral pleural
effusion, marked pulmonary vascular congestion, and an enlarged heart;
the basilar portions of both lungs were deaerated by fluid compression.

Laboratory studies
Hemoglobin and hematocrit—within normal limits.
Serum sodium level—at the upper limits of normal.
Potassium—3.2 mEq./L. (normal, 3.5 to 5).
Chloride—94 mEq./L. (normal, 96 to 105).
pH—7.5 (7.35 to 7.45).
A slightly elevated BUN, 50 mg./100 ml. (normal, 10 to 20), and a lowered
creatinine clearance, 46 ml./min. (normal, 70 to 130), suggest some im-
pairment in renal function.
Urinalysis—within normal limits.

Medical therapy
The physician's plan of *medical therapy* included:
    Sodium restriction.
    Fluid restriction.
    Acid-base balance with diuretics.
    Maximize digitalis effects.
    Consider thoracentesis and paracentesis.
The physician's *immediate orders* were as follows:
    1000 mg. of sodium diet.
    Restrict fluids to 1000 ml./day.
    Up to bathroom.
    Up in chair, ad lib.
    Vital signs t.i.d.
    Intake and output.
    Daily weights.
    Elastic stockings.
    Bedboard.
    O_2 via nasal prongs at 2 L./min. p.r.n.
    Medications:
        Digoxin, 0.25 mg., q.d.
        Isosorbide dinitrate (Iordil), 5 mg., p.o., q.i.d.

Nitroglycerin, 0.6 mg., no. 5 at bedside.

Darvon Compound, 65 mg., p.o., q.4h., p.r.n.

Secobarbital (Seconal), 50 mg., p.o., q.h., p.r.n.

Furosemide (Lasix), 160 mg., p.o. every morning.

20% KCl, 10 ml. p.o., b.i.d.

Dioctyl sodium sulfosuccinate (Colace), 100 mg., p.o. b.i.d.

Spironolactone (Aldactone A), 25 mg., p.o., q.d.

Mr. Hunt became progressively more dyspneic on his arrival to the division. He appeared restless and apprehensive. He seemed to become increasingly demanding on nursing time for physical and emotional care and increasingly more difficult to please. Within an hour of his arrival, Mr. Hunt was transferred to a private room to facilitate his rest.

The physician was called to evaluate Mr. Hunt's increasing respiratory distress and ordered the following *drugs to be given immediately* to facilitate respiratory and cardiac function:

Furosemide, 80 mg., p.o., immediately.

Morphine sulfate, 3 mg., subcutaneously.

Aminophyllin suppositories, 500 mg., per rectum.

Ammonium chloride, 2 Gm., p.o.

20% KCl, 10 ml. p.o.

Oxygen at 3 L.

Diazepam (Valium), 10 mg., p.o.

A thoracentesis was done about 8:00 P.M., and approximately 700 ml. of fluid was removed from the pleural cavity. This fluid was analyzed in the laboratory and found not to contain malignant cells or any bacteria.

Based upon the assessment of the patient, a plan was made for the first 24 hours of Mr. Hunt's care. The main objectives were to help bring into balance the demand for oxygen supply and carbon dioxide removal and to reduce the stress on the heart. These objectives were met by (1) reducing requirements of the body for oxygen, (2) increasing cardiac output, and (3) eliminating edema.

NURSING CARE PLAN

GOALS	NURSING INTERVENTIONS
Reduce cellular demands for oxygen and CO_2 transport.	Transfer to private room. Put electric bed in lowest position.
Reduce motor activity.	Encourage to stay in bed except to go to the bathroom.
Promote physical and emotional comfort.	Call central switchboard and restrict telephone calls to immediate family. Restrict visitors to one at a time for only 2 or 3 min.

Continued.

NURSING CARE PLAN—cont'd

GOALS	NURSING INTERVENTIONS
	Try to meet requests as made by Mr. Hunt.
	Reassure that nurse will be checking on him every 10 minutes.
	Pin bell cord to pillow; show him where it is.
	Make sure wrist watch is wound and has accurate time.
	Explain procedures in terms of what the nurse is going to do, what the doctor will be doing, and what he is to do.
	Give bed bath.
	Monitor vital signs q.6h. (BP, T.P.R.); notify doctor if systolic pressure is less than 100; after thoracentesis, monitor BP, P.R., q.½h. twice, q.1h. twice, q.2h. twice, q.4h. until morning.
	Record pulse and respiratory rate before and after activity (for example, going to bathroom, eating).
	Record any anginal pain and when nitroglycerin taken.
	Plan rest periods between each nursing care or patient activity.
	Instruct to call for assistance to go to bathroom; encourage standing to void, with use of urinal at bedside.
	Avoid, if possible, giving diuretics after 6:00 P.M.
	Give secobarbital, 50 mg., p.o., at 10:00 P.M.
	Give warm milk with sedative.
	Place sheepskin under Mr. Hunt.
Promote ventilatory expansion.	Head of bed elevated at 45 degrees or position of comfort.
	Support arms with pillows.
	Encourage turning side to back to side q.1h.
	Oxygen by nasal prongs at 2 L./min.; record response to oxygen; place small cotton ball under each side of nasal prong to relieve pressure at side of head.
	Be sure humidifier is filled; check q.4h.
	Encourage to breathe as deeply as possible and to cough q.1h. to raise secretions.
Reduce cardiac work load and circulatory volume:	Give diuretic and cardiac drugs as ordered by physician.
	Weigh daily before breakfast in pajamas only; use same scale each day.
Participate in diuretic therapy.	Record intake and output accurately each shift.
	Measure abdominal girth q.d. before breakfast.
Restrict fluids.	Remove elastic stockings q.4h. for 15 min.; reapply.
Give 1000 mg. sodium diet.	Restrict oral fluids to 1000 ml./day: 500 ml. for day shift, 300 ml. for evening shift, and 200 ml. for night shift.
	Give fluids that may be cool or at room temperature.
	Talk to dietitian about coordinating fluids with meals and medications.

NURSING CARE PLAN—cont'd

GOALS	NURSING INTERVENTIONS
	Encourage not to strain while having a bowel movement.
	Record consistency of stool.
	Give Colace, 100 mg., p.o., at 8:00 A.M. and 6:00 P.M.
Encourage ingestion of nutrients to meet physiologic needs.	Arrange for dietitian to talk to patient regarding food preferences.
	Arrange with dietitian to include warm milk at h.s. within sodium and fluid restrictions.
	May feed himself.
	Arrange with dietary department for small between-meal snacks.
	Position comfortably in order to facilitate eating; open milk carton, remove covers, etc. to spare energy for eating.
	Observe and record nutritional intake.
	Observe patient for increasing symptoms of anorexia or gastrointestinal disturbances—often an early sign of drug toxicity.
	Rinse mouth before meals with half-strength mouthwash solution.
	Soak dentures in cleansing solution brought from home.

RESPONSE TO NURSING INTERVENTION

Mr. Hunt responded dramatically to his therapy during the first 48 hours. He no longer required oxygen for ease of respiration; his respiratory rate decreased to 20 at rest with no discomfort or effort. His repeat chest films showed a resolution of pulmonary edema. His repeat ECG showed a digitalis effect, regular beats, and left ventricular hypertrophy. Mr. Hunt's weight dropped from 70.3 kg. (154.6 lb.) to 58.2 kg. (128 lb.), his abdominal girth dropped from 40.2 inches to 36 inches, indicating a decrease in his ascites and hepatomegaly. His fluid restrictions were removed.

Mr. Hunt continued to be a "difficult patient to please." Some of the problems were resolved by following a fairly rigid schedule, allowing rest periods between each activity:

Morning:

8:00, Weight, in pajamas.

8:30-9:00, Breakfast.

10:00, Assist with bath; wash back and legs.

11:00-11:30, In chair with legs elevated.

Afternoon:
  12:30-1:00, Lunch.
  2:00, Walk in hall to nurses' station.
  6:00-6:30, Dinner.
  7:30, Walk in hall to nurses' station.
  10:00, Bedtime care.
  10:30, Medications.

Mr. Hunt also appreciated having the nurse in charge stop by frequently to ask him how he was doing and what he would like to have done for him.

Mr. Hunt was an alert, responsive gentleman who seemed to have some understanding of his cardiac illness. He was able to relate exertion and emotional upset to his anginal pain, and a low-salt diet to reducing edema. The physician planned on sending Mr. Hunt home on his current medication regime. The nursing care plan was altered to prepare Mr. Hunt to return home.

MODIFIED NURSING CARE PLAN

GOALS	NURSING INTERVENTIONS
Gradually increase activity to meet his activity requirements at home.	Encourage patient to give own morning care. Gradually allow him to assume total responsibility for personal hygiene. Continue to monitor and record pulse, respiration, and fatigue after activity. Help Mr. Hunt plan for frequent rest periods during day in hospital and at home.
Teach him to take his own medications.	Show him each medication at each time of administration; explain the action of each medication. Help him plan a way to remember to take the medication and when to take it.
Encourage regular medical care.	Encourage him to keep regular appointments with physician. Encourage him to weigh himself daily and keep a record. Have him notify physician if he notices any increase in fatigue, in shortness of breath, or in weight. Have him notify physician if he notices any increase in loss of appetite, in nausea, or in other gastrointestinal symptoms.
Help him to meet dietary needs and to follow restrictions.	Talk with nurse/housekeeper when she visits to determine whether sodium restriction has been followed and ways sodium may be reduced. Plan with Mr. Hunt ways he may follow dietary restrictions when he is out for dinner (for example, order fruit plates and plain foods; never add salt to foods; ask to have salt eliminated from preparation of a broiled meat).

Ten days after admission, Mr. Hunt's condition was so much improved that he was allowed to go home. At this time he was ambulatory and able to care for most of his own needs.

CHAPTER 11

POSTOPERATIVE NEEDS OF A MAN HAVING OPEN-HEART SURGERY

MARJORIE ROTT

MEDICAL HISTORY

"Little did I think, 18 months ago, that I would have to come to this huge, confusing big-city medical center for a complicated operation, when I just felt so tired and short of breath," reflected Mr. Walter Evans. Upon admission to a medical-surgical unit of single rooms at this center, Mr. Evans identified that it was because of "heart trouble" that his local physician had referred him here for definitive care. Mr. Evans recounted having rheumatic fever when he was 13 years old and hinted at the frustration of having to stay in bed for several months and miss outdoor activities with school friends. Although left with a heart murmur, he had no limitation of activities. He was in good general health until 18 months prior to this admission, when he experienced dyspnea on exertion. At that time, he was hospitalized by his local physician, diagnosed as having aortic stenosis, and treated successfully with digitalis and diuretics. He returned to his usual activities on maintenance medications until 2 months prior to admission when dyspnea was evident upon climbing one flight of stairs and "increasing nervousness" accompanied his shortness of breath. Admission to the medical center had been planned for diagnostic cardiac catheterization on March 14 to determine the degree of cardiac impairment, but admission was necessitated earlier, on March 5, because of Mr. Evans' increasing discomfort.

Physical examination, on admission, revealed the following pertinent data about Mr. Evans: height, 6 feet; weight, 78.3 kg.; oral temperature, 36.6° C. (97.9° F.); apical pulse, 70 per minute and irregularly irregular; quiet, even respirations at 18 per minute at rest with good expansion and excursion of the chest, but with scattered rales bilaterally at the lung bases; blood pressure at rest was 118/70. A systolic murmur was audible across the chest, radiating to the right neck and left axillary regions. There was no neck-vein distension or peripheral edema; pedal pulses were palpable as soft and equal.

PSYCHOSOCIAL BACKGROUND

A 49-year-old white male, Mr. Evans has been married for 30 years and lives with his wife and two of their four children who are still at home. He completed high school, plumber's trade requirements, and worked for 25 years as an independent plumber in their small home town 50 miles from here. Five years ago, he began working as a salesman for a plumbing supply firm, which requires occasional 1-day trips. He enjoys gardening and home remodeling projects and watching local high school and professional sports. His wife seemed tense and quiet, deferring to her husband for interpretation of questions.

MEDICAL EVALUATION

Medical plans during the preoperative evaluation stage of Mr. Evans' hospitalization included the following:

Digoxin, 0.25 mg., p.o., q.d.

Ethacrynic acid (Edecrin), 50 mg., p.o., q.d.

Diazepam (Valium), 5 mg., p.o., t.i.d.

Secobarbital (Seconal), 0.1 Gm., p.o., q.h.s., p.r.n.

1500 ml. fluid, q.d. limit.

Intake and output.

Weigh q.d. before breakfast.

Blood value determinations showed that Mr. Evans' BUN, electrolytes, and FBS were within the normal ranges as were his hematocrit at 45 vol.%, and WBC at 8000 mm.[3]. His prothrombin time was 70% to 85% of normal. His electrocardiogram showed an irregularly irregular QRS rhythm without P waves—atrial fibrillation and left ventricular hypertrophy. Chest X-ray film demonstrated left ventricular cardiac enlargement and congestive changes in both lungs, but with no evidence of present interalveolar or interstitial edema. The enlarged left ventricle was also noted on X-ray views of the heart during a barium swallow procedure. When the chest was examined under fluoroscopy, cardiomegaly was evident, with calcification of the aortic valve.

NURSING ASSESSMENT AND PREOPERATIVE TEACHING

During several days of physical examination by the cardiac surgical team and medical cardiologist, Miss Harte (one of the clinical nurses) was establishing a relationship with Mr. Evans and was identifying and planning to meet his nursing care requirements. She had begun her evaluation when she admitted him to the division, noting his restlessness and repeated questions about timing of doctors' visits, examinations, tests, visiting hours, etc. She explained the hospital daily schedule, and each day personnel stopped during morning rounds to explain what he could expect during that day. Miss Harte waited each time and offered her assistance with any further questions. As X-ray examination and other tests were completed, the physicians were able to tell Mr. Evans the nature of the "narrowed heart valve" and their recommendations for surgical replacement. Remembering his general nervousness with diagnostic procedures and that Mr. Evans had been hospitalized only once before for the treatment of his first onset of dyspnea, Miss Harte assessed his need for preoperative instruction. Understanding that moderate anxiety is better worked through by specific information given preoperatively, Miss Harte planned a time with him to discuss the sequence of events associated with surgery. She sat down with him and offered an outline of events—skin preparation; medications; waking up in the recovery room with oxygen, intravenous, and chest tubes inserted; the close availability of nursing personnel and pain medication to assist in the important postoperative movement, coughing, and lung reexpansion. He was quiet, but asked about how much pain he would have and how long the surgery and recovery room time would be. She answered in specific terms—pain would be relieved to a tolerable level with medication; he would be asleep most of the day, and then after being awake for an hour or so, he would be transferred from the recovery room to the intensive care unit. Mr. Evans seemed satisfied and stated that he would explain this to his wife. He was visited by the Catholic chaplain who explained that he would be back that evening to give last rites. Last rites are routinely given to patients undergoing cardiac surgery.

On the day before surgery, Miss Sawyer from the intensive care unit came to interview Mr. Evans. Miss Harte offered her assessment of him and shared with Miss Sawyer the schedule of information-giving she had planned for him. (See teaching summary.) During her interview with Mr. Evans, Miss Sawyer answered his specific questions about how long he would be in the unit, how much pain he would have, and when his family could visit. She listed for him some of the things that would occur—frequent taking of temperature, pulse, and blood pressure; the use of oxygen, the intermittent positive pressure breathing (IPPB) machine, and intravenous fluids. She had him demonstrate coughing and deep-breathing exercises he had learned and showed him shoulder range of motion. She noted that his general color was pale, but that his lips and nailbeds were pink and that his pedal pulses were faint and equal in volume. She talked with Miss Harte about his comments concerning other postoperative cardiac surgery patients, his fear of "coughing being the most painful part" and his jovial manner, which may have been an indication of anxiety. She indicated she would plan his immediate postoperative care with the other intensive care unit nurses and promised to keep the family and the floor nurses up to date on his progress.

PREOPERATIVE TEACHING SUMMARY

DATA	GOAL	NURSING INTERVENTIONS
49 years old. High school graduate. Plumbing supply sales- man. Preoperative for aortic valve replacement on March 10. Restless; pacing in room. Repeats questions. "Difficulty breathing when nervous." Married, 4 children. Catholic.	Offer preoperative teach- ing in small amounts with specific informa- tion to minimize anx- iety and to introduce skills needed post- operatively.	Give information ½ to 1 day prior to events. Offer chance for him to ask questions. Give factual answers to questions asked. On March 6, give specific information regarding his participation in bar- ium swallow and car- diac fluoroscopy; ex- plain 1500 ml. fluid re- striction—pitcher at bedside marked 700 ml., with 800 ml. to come with meals. On March 8, offer step- by-step description of preoperative and recov- ery room procedures; demonstrate deep breathing and cough- ing; Mr. Evans should return demonstration once during the day and once during the evening. On March 9, introduce to intensive care nurse; practice coughing, deep breathing, and use of IPPB machine; discuss family visiting hours; routine of last rites from priest before surgery.

SURGERY

Mr. Evans' preanesthetic medication was morphine sulfate, 10 mg., and scopolamine, 0.4 mg., I.M., 1½ hours prior to going to the operating room. There he received thiopental sodium intravenously to induce anesthesia and was maintained on nitrous oxide, oxygen, and halothane via an oral endotracheal tube during the 6-hour procedure. After Mr. Evans' cardiac and respiratory functions were transferred to the bypass pump oxygenator, the surgical team replaced his calcified aortic valve with a Starr-Edwards prosthetic aortic valve. Two thoracotomy tubes were inserted and the sternal incision was closed. The endotracheal tube was left in place, oxygen was supplied, and Mr. Evans was transferred to the recovery room with the following medical notations:

Postoperative aortic valve replacement for aortic stenosis.

Condition: Satisfactory.

Vital signs: P, R, and BP q.15min. until stable, then q.½h. 8 times; central venous pressure (CVP) and T. q.1h.

O_2 at 6 L./min.

Activity: Bed rest tonight.

Head of bed at 30 degrees elevation if BP and P remain stable.

Progressive ambulation in A.M. as tolerated.

Diet: N.P.O. for 6 hours; then fluids as tolerated and progress to 1500 mg. sodium diet.

Thoracotomy tubes to -30 cm. H_2O pressure.

Replace drainage milliliter for milliliter with whole blood (right arm).

I.V. 5% dextrose in water (right groin), 80 ml./h.

(I.V. and p.o. to 2000 ml./day).

Foley catheter to closed drainage.

Intake and output q.1h.

Oxacillin, 1 Gm., q.6h., I.V. (500 mg., p.o. q.6h. when taking diet) for 10 days.

Streptomycin, 500 mg., q.12h., I.M. for 5 days.

Laboratory work stat and in morning: ECG, chest X-ray film, hematocrit, electrolytes, blood gases.

POSTOPERATIVE CARE

In the immediate postoperative period, Mr. Evans was lethargic but responded to his name and simple directions to turn. His pulse ranged from 70 to 110; respirations, 14 to 20; blood pressure, 90 to 120/palpable; CVP, 18 to 20 cm. H_2O pressure.

The following medications were ordered to treat beginning congestive heart failure and possible fluid overload:

Lanatoside C (Cedilanid), 0.2 mg., I.V.

Ethacrynic acid (Edecrin), 50 mg., I.V., q.6h. 3 times.

Furosemide (Lasix), 40 mg., I.V.

Mr. Evans' CVP gradually stabilized between 8 and 12 cm. H_2O; pulse, irregular at 70 to 80; blood pressure, audible at $\frac{100\text{-}120}{60\text{-}70}$. His urine output ranged between 25 and 75 ml./h. He was given morphine, 6 mg., subcutaneously, as he became restless with gradually increasing awareness of discomfort. He was suctioned occasionally through the endotracheal tube, and his breath sounds were audible clearly over all lobes. As he became more alert and was able to breathe more comfortably and deeply with pain relief, the endotracheal tube was removed and oxygen was supplied by a nasal pronged catheter. After 4 hours in the recovery room, Mr. Evans was transferred to the intensive care unit, where his family was able to see him for a short period.

NURSING CARE IN THE INTENSIVE CARE UNIT

During the first night Mr. Evans' vital signs, thoracotomy drainage, and urine output were monitored frequently. He was turned and repositioned every hour with the thoracotomy tubes held stable to minimize pain. Morphine was given every 3 or 4 hours, and Mr. Evans was required to deep-breathe and cough every hour. Encouragement and assistance was offered by the nurse, who splinted both sides of his incision with her hands and applied counterpressure on exhalation to stimulate coughing and stabilize the chest incision.

Mr. Evans appeared pale and slightly dusky and developed slight nasal flaring and supraclavicular retraction during this first postoperative night. The physicians were notified of this and were informed that his breath sounds were less clear and that his cough continued to be nonproductive. Treatments to humidify the air passages and liquefy secretions with mechanically forced deep inspiration were begun:

Ultrasonic nebulizer for 5 min. q.4h.

IPPB at 15 cm. H_2O pressure with 2 ml. Mucomyst and 2 ml. normal saline for 7 to 10 min. q.4h.

Miss Sawyer explained and demonstrated these mechanical aids to deep breathing and removal of mucus secretions. She offered pain medication prior to the treatments and coughing, and Mr. Evans agreed to "try the gadgets" and cough harder.

He was quite fatigued from the frequent interruptions during the night and had "knifelike" incisional pain. His temperature had gradually risen to 39.5° C. (103.1° F.) rectally by noon. After a morning rest period, he was able to sit with the head of the bed rolled up and to take liquids at noon.

By planning the spacing of rest and activity periods and by giving pain medication before the necessary activities of postoperative care, the staff was able to achieve the nursing care goals set for Mr. Evans. After the second IPPB treatment, he was able to cough out plugs of thick mucus and was breathing without effort or rib retraction. These treatments were continued on an every 4-hour basis for 2 days until his temperature was 37.5° C. (99.5° F.) to 38.5° C. (101.3° F.) orally and his chest X-ray film showed "evidence of resolving atelectasis." The schedule was then decreased to four times a day, with the night activities limited to every 3- to 4-hour turning with back care, coughing, deep breathing, and vital sign monitoring. This allowed longer periods of natural sleep after several days of sleep deprivation.

During these first few days, Mr. Evans was gradually able to be more active. The first morning he dangled his legs over the edge of the bed, and that evening he was up in a chair for 5 minutes with the thoracotomy tubes clamped and the groin I.V. removed. After the thoracotomy tubes were removed on the second day, he was up for gradually longer and more frequent periods. He was taking fluids and a soft diet without difficulty, and his arm I.V. tubing was removed on the third morning.

Mr. Evans continued to cough shallowly despite the use of pain medication and coaching and encouragement from the staff. He seemed to "hold back" and appeared apprehensive about this activity. A low-grade fever and X-ray signs of right lower-lobe atelectasis persisted. He occasionally complained of shortness of breath and discomfort when requested to do coughing and deep-breathing exercises. A physical therapist was consulted; she discussed the need for these activities with Mr. Evans and developed the following modifications with him, the physicians, and the nurses:

1. Schedule respiratory therapies midway between meals when the stomach is not full of food or fluids.
2. Continue to use pain medication prior to treatments (Mr. Evans is fearful about "anticipated" pain).
3. Start Mr. Evans with blow bottles to have him gradually increase his inspiratory and expiratory single breaths "at his own pace."
4. After he has "limbered up," have him use the IPPB machine, which will effect greater inspiratory volumes and depth with nebulization of the liquefying agent, Alevaire.
5. Help him to support his own incision with a pillow and direct him to cough against his own support. (He seemed to feel more confident when he could take an active part in minimizing the discomfort of this treatment.)

This plan was carried out by the nursing staff, and Mr. Evans gradually was able to cough more deeply with somewhat less apprehension and discomfort.

Mr. Evans' strength and general comfort gradually increased. He had occasional rises in temperature late in the day and periodic diaphoretic episodes. His cough continued to produce thick white, occasionally gray, mucus. He was able to do the "upper half" of his bath, to turn by himself in bed, and to get out of bed with the assistance of one person.

On the fourth postoperative day, he was to be transferred back to his original medical-surgical unit; Miss Sawyer summarized his postoperative course to give the nurses on the unit adequate data to meet Mr. Evans' needs in a way that would ease the transition for him.

TRANSITION TO CONVALESCENT UNIT

After receiving a report from Miss Sawyer on Mr. Evans' postoperative course in the intensive care unit, Miss Harte began to plan for his continued nursing care on the general unit. As she helped him get settled in his room, she was assessing his general responses to her greeting and questions and was noting his strength and ability to move about, his facial and peripheral color, his respiratory rate and depth, and his pulse rate, rhythm, and volume. She reviewed his medical orders, the physicians' estimate of discharge in 7 to 10 days after resolution of the residual atelectasis. Miss Harte then wrote out a "working care plan of priorities" to assist the nursing staff in continuing Mr. Evans' postoperative care. The purposes of this action were to provide consistency in care that would ease his transition from the intensive care setting to the convalescent unit and to reassess and adjust his care to meet his changing requirements.

POSTOPERATIVE PRIORITIES CARE PLAN

DATA	GOAL	NURSING INTERVENTIONS

Respiratory:
  Shallow cough, occasionally productive.
  "Retained secretions."
  "Resolving right lower lobe atelectasis."
Incisional pain.
Low-grade fever.
Periodic diaphoresis.
	Maximize coughing to remove secretions and resolve atelectasis.
	Maximize comfort.
		Offer pain medication prior to blow bottles and IPPB.
		Stay with him during treatments—scheduled midway between meals.
		Provide pillow for him to hold during deep breathing and coughing—remind him with hand pressure to cough during exhalation.
		Assist with bath—assemble items and wash back and legs.

Continued.

POSTOPERATIVE PRIORITIES CARE PLAN—cont'd

DATA	GOAL	NURSING INTERVENTIONS
		Leave several changes of hospital pajamas each morning; offer to change bed linen as necessary.
		Check midafternoon and evening for wet linen.
Cardiac-fluid balance: Slightly pale. Pulse irregular, strong 70-80. Incision healing. "Up ad lib"—walk in hall at least q.i.d. 2000 ml. fluid limit. 1500 mg. sodium diet. Maintenance warfarin, 5 mg., q.d.	Continue supervision of vital signs, weight, intake and output, and medications. Provide useful information for home care: activity, diet, medications.	See Kardex for schedule of vital signs, medications, etc. (March 15) Help him to get out of bed; accompany him in hall until stable. Review understanding of digitalis, furosemide, schedules, untoward symptoms. Assess knowledge of high-sodium foods, previous diet planning, fluid allotment spacing (refer to dietitian if indicated), action of warfarin, and need for periodic blood tests.
Emotional: "General fatigue and discomfort"; fearful about continued pain; occasionally mentions: "How long will it be before I can go gack to work?" "Sleeping poorly." Likes Sanka at h.s.	Evaluate items of concern to him. Maximize postoperative recovery and resumption of activities.	Assess understanding of "gradually progressing activities for 4 to 6 weeks at home, and then gradually resume work responsibilities." Provide specific periods when nurse is available to talk with him and/or discuss questions. (9:00-10:00 P.M.) Offer Sanka and pain medication; change or straighten linen as necessary; back rub after coughing and range-of-motion exercises.

POSTOPERATIVE PRIORITIES CARE PLAN—cont'd

DATA	GOAL	NURSING INTERVENTIONS
		Do not awaken during night for vital signs unless 8:00 P.M. temperature elevated.

CHAPTER 12

A WOMAN REQUIRING PERIPHERAL VASCULAR SURGERY

NANCY GORENSHEK

MEDICAL HISTORY

Mrs. Grace Jones, a black 56-year-old widow, was admitted to the hospital with numbness and increasing coolness of her right foot over the past several months. She gives a history of having injured this leg 8 months earlier. After the injury, an ulcer developed on the lower portion of the tibia. Mrs. Jones has had mild diabetes for the past 5 years and had been started on tolbutamide (Orinase) tablets several times a day, but discontinued the drug without medical advice. Her physician also diagnosed hypertension, but she did not take any of the medication he prescribed for it.

On admission, Mrs. Jones' fasting blood sugar was 250 mg./100 ml. (normal, 65 to 110). Other blood chemistries were within normal limits.

PSYCHOSOCIAL BACKGROUND

Mrs. Jones was born in Alabama and is presently living alone in a 4½-room first-floor apartment in a large midwestern city. She receives $94 per month from her husband's Social Security benefits, and supplements this by doing domestic work 2 or 3 days a week. Since the death of her husband several years ago, a cousin and a neighbor have been helpful to her at times when she has been under stress. The neighbor volunteered to care for her apartment during her hospitalization.

SURGICAL INTERVENTION

The arteriograms performed shortly after Mrs. Jones' admission to the hospital showed multiple arteriosclerotic plaque formation throughout the entire femoral artery and a complete block of the popliteal artery just above the knee joint. The anterior tibial, perineal, and posterior tibial arteries were filled by collateral circulation, and these arteries had irregular plaque formation and narrowing by arteriosclerosis. After the diagnosis was made, Mrs. Jones was taken to surgery for a femoral-popliteal bypass operation, using the saphenous vein for the graft. A debridement and graft of the lower right leg ulcer was also completed, using skin from the left thigh for this graft.

NURSING INTERVENTION

After surgery, Mrs. Jones' right leg began to swell and was slightly warmer than the unaffected extremity. Hyperemia is a result of increased vascularization and therefore increased metabolic activities that occur in a once-ischemic area. Her right leg was elevated on pillows to facilitate venous return and lymphatic drainage. A linen guard (cradle) was also placed on the bed to prevent pressure on the affected limb and to decrease disruption of the skin graft. She was encouraged to keep her right leg as straight as possible, thereby eliminating pressure on the graft.

Mrs. Jones' lower extremities were wrapped firmly and evenly with elastic bandages to assist in compression of the superficial vessels and to aid in venous return. A careful assessment of her circulation was made through frequent checks of the tibial and pedal pulses and through observations of color and temperature changes. This was done to ensure that circulation was adequate and that emboli were not present.

When she ambulated, Mrs. Jones was helped to keep her right leg extended. Sitting was discouraged because it would interfere with venous return. Since nylon stockings with elastic tops could also cause a disturbance in venous return, Mrs. Jones was advised not to wear this kind of stocking.

Shortly after her operations, plans were begun for Mrs. Jones' homegoing. These plans included instruction about the prescribed diabetic diet, foot care, and self-medication. She was to take tolbutamide, methyldopa (Aldomet), and ferrous sulfate daily. A referral was made to the Visiting Nurse Association requesting the services of a nurse who would visit her at home, evaluate her ability to care for herself, and assist with dressing changes on her right leg. Since Mrs. Jones had discontinued her medications prior to hospitalization, it was important to have someone check with her at home to be sure she was taking the medications as ordered. Additional arrangements included a follow-up visit to the surgical outpatient clinic 4 weeks after discharge from the hospital. She would then be followed in the diabetic clinic.

CHAPTER 13

A TEEN-AGER WITH CHRONIC RENAL FAILURE

JEANETTE BALDWIN

MEDICAL HISTORY

Betty is an 18-year-old female who has had 22 hospital admissions, beginning with an admission diagnosis of subacute glomerulonephritis when she was 9 years old. When she was admitted to the renal unit, her diagnoses were acute renal failure secondary to chronic renal failure, congestive heart disease, and hypertension. She has had 9 years of progressive renal disease, repeated hospitalizations, conservative medical treatment, and numerous peritoneal dialyses.

Until this admission her total physiologic condition was in a state of relative balance for 9 months. She has been on a 2 Gm. sodium and 40 Gm. protein diet. Her fluid restriction has varied with her salt retention, but usually was maintained at 1000 ml. per 24 hours. Since she has had persistent edema not subsiding with rest and dietary regimen, she has been taking hydrochlorothiazide (HydroDiuril), 50 mg., q.d. Although treated with methyldopa (Aldomet), 500 mg., q.i.d., and hydralazine (Apresoline), 50 mg., q.i.d., her blood pressure has fluctuated between 150/90 and 210/120. She has been treated vigorously three times in the last 3 years for congestive heart failure and associated pulmonary edema. There is no family history of kidney disease. Two siblings and her mother are healthy. Her father has mild hypertension associated with obesity. After treatment of her renal crisis, Betty is to be evaluated for continued medical management, maintenance hemodialysis, or renal transplantation.

PSYCHOSOCIAL BACKGROUND

During the last 9 years, Betty has attended school regularly. She has been graduated from high school and has earned a scholarship at a state university. Certainly her record indicates a positive intellectual environment as does her psychologic testing. There are many potential sources of strength in this patient's interpersonal, sociocultural, and spiritual environments. Her mother and father, both in their forties, work full time and seem to have a close relationship with

74

Betty and with each other. Her sister, a senior in high school, does many things with Betty, and her brother, a sophomore, relates normally to Betty. She has few close friends, but has a strong family constellation of grandparents, aunts, uncles, and cousins. She draws a great deal of support from two of her former teachers (nuns) and uses them as reference points. Betty has, of course, known many doctors and health workers, but has had the same medical nephrologist for the last 3 years. His medical therapeutic plan includes the imparting to her of information about her present and future medical status. She has always been deemed a "good patient" by health personnel and a "good child" by her significant figures. As will be documented later, the problems of "good patients" are often hidden behind a cloak of conformity.

MEDICAL THERAPY

Bed rest for the congestive heart failure.

Rapid digitalization.

Rotating tourniquets.

Vigorous diuretic therapy.

Adequate pulmonary ventilation.

Hemodialysis for 8 hours after the clinical and biochemical determination of uremia: nausea, coma, hyperkalemia, and intense catabolic reaction.

Resumption of the conservative medical regimen after stabilization of renal function, cardiac, and pulmonary status.

Renal biopsy and electron microscopy.

Transfusion with one unit of fresh blood (hematocrit: 16 vol.% [normal range, 37 to 47 vol.%]).

Social, psychiatric, and urologic consultations regarding feasibility of renal transplant.

Evaluation of mother as potential kidney donor.

NURSING OBJECTIVES

Monitor fluids and electrolyte body balance and intervene when necessary to ensure stabilization of the internal environment of the body.

With any acute or chronic renal disease, imbalances likely to occur are metabolic acidosis, potassium excess, fluid balance excess, and/or calcium excess. In addition, administration of potent diuretics can precipitate a sodium deficit. On admission, Betty was immediately placed on a Brookline metabolic scale. If this were not available, a bed scale could have been used. Accurate weights are easier to obtain for patients with renal failure than accurate outputs, and rapid variations in weight can closely reflect changes in fluid volume. During Betty's hemodialysis, she lost 2 kg. in 1 hour, which being accompanied by a drop in blood pressure from 160/110 to 80/20, prompted the nurse to begin a saline intravenous drip and to notify the physician. As Betty regained renal function gradually, a 0.2 kg. daily weight gain reflected improved metabolism rather than fluid retention.

Vital signs (T.P.R. and BP) reflect changes in body imbalance. Initially, Betty's temperature of 39° C. (102.2° F.) may have been indicative of infection, or possibly of sodium excess. After 4 hours of hemodialysis, weak, irregular, rapid pulse (from 102 to 126), as well as her ECG rhythm, indicated severe potassium deficit. These improved after potassium was administered. Since metabolic acidosis affects the rate and depth of breathing by greatly increasing both, it is important to observe breathing for a full 2 minutes. Occasionally Betty's vital signs were checked by auxiliary personnel, following specific instructions given to them by the registered nurse. Of course, skin elasticity and mucous membrane moisture are important indices and were of help in determining Betty's fluid-volume excess. Although some muscle twitching was present, her blood calcium level was normal. As the medical regimen controlled Betty's initial acute renal failure, close measurement of intake and output as well as daily weights assumed importance in assessing renal function. Daily serum levels of sodium (134 to 145 mEq./L.), potassium (3.5 to 5 mEq./L.), chloride (96 to 105 mEq./L.), and pH (7.35 to 7.45) were used to monitor the chemical homeostasis of the body. A serum sodium of 156 mEq./L. one day reflected the potato chips Betty had eaten. It is simple to check the pH of the urine frequently, and depending on her food and sleep patterns, Betty's pH usually was 4.5 (normal, 4.5 to 7.5), indicating a tendency toward acidosis.

Physiologically assess the patient holistically as well as in terms of renal dysfunction; in chronic renal disease, all organ systems are interrelated in delicate balance.

Renal dysfunction is, of course, assessed by nursing history, physical observation, examination of the urine, blood chemistries, and tests of glomerular and tubular function. Betty's urine specific gravity was 1.006 (normal, 1.010 to 1.025). This low value is consistent with chronic renal disease and decreased ability to concentrate urine and a low-protein and low-salt diet. A urine specific gravity is simple to perform and tells much about the patient's entire physiologic status. Betty's diuresis, resulting from administration of diuretics and hemodialysis, lowered the specific gravity of her urine. Determination of the urinary pH, glucose, and albumin can be made at the bedside. Betty's urine showed the presence of albumin, later confirmed chemically by a urinary urea nitrogen of 68 Gm. per 24 hours (normal, 5 to 13 Gm.). Elevation of the blood urea nitrogen is a well-documented sign of renal insufficiency. Usually the serum creatinine parallels the BUN, although authorities disagree somewhat on the validity of differential elevation of BUN and creatinine. Betty's initial BUN was 158 mg./100 ml. (normal, 10 to 20) and creatinine, 16 mg./100 ml. (normal, 0.7 to 1.2). After 10 hours on the Kiil dialyzer, her BUN stabilized at 53 and creatinine at 11. The most accurate test of glomerular function or measurement of glomerular filtration rate is the determination of creatinine clearance. This simple measurement was done daily for Betty and averaged 20 to 25 ml./min. (normal, 70 to 130). A urine concentration test was not done since her renal tubular reabsorption was minimal on previous admissions.

Headaches are a common symptom of renal disease, particularly since hypertension accompanies primary renal dysfunction. Betty's headaches were caused in part, too, by a shift in fluid and electrolytes resulting from diuretic administration, antihypertensives, and hemodialysis. She had a shift from an elevated to a lower serum sodium and from an acid pH to alkalosis. In addition, she lost 4 kg. in 24 hours. Her edema was generally periorbital and caused by renal retention of sodium and water. Signs of cerebral edema were not present. Anemia, more severe with a high degree of azotemia, can contribute to the development of congestive heart failure and acidosis. With an initial hematocrit of 16 vol.% (normal, 37 to 47), Betty was given two units of whole blood and her hematocrit stabilized at 21. Since her potassium was high, stored blood was not used. Because stored red blood cells still contain viable enzymes, a certain amount of metabolism occurs, releasing potassium by hemolysis. Mild bleeding of her gums occurred in the beginning and was associated with anemia. Betty's pruritus and dry skin (possibly symptomatic of early uremia) were relieved by antipruritic lotions and baths. Caladryl lotion and triamcinolone acetonide (Kenalog), 0.025% spray, were effective as were Alpha-Keri baths. Since a low resistance to infection accompanies renal failure, observation for urinary tract infections particularly, as well as for pneumonitis and septicemia is important. The nurse's role in assessment is to observe, analyze, determine significant relationships, and utilize scientific physiologic principles, as well as logical processes as rationale for making valid judgments about appropriate nursing intervention.

Sustain the patient during the acute crisis psychologically as well as physiologically.

During her initial 8 hours and during her 10 hours of hemodialysis, Betty needed mostly supportive care—help in conserving her energy. Emotional support encompassed letting her know that someone would stay with her, that the person can be trusted, and in general terms, what is being done for her and why. Betty was encouraged to verbalize her concerns. The patient's fear of the unknown and the presence of strange equipment and many medical personnel require that the nurse provide explanations and opportunities for the patient to verbalize her thoughts and feelings. Often the nurse was a sounding board or gave simple answers to short questions.

Plan, test out, and evaluate nursing interventions to help the patient mobilize her resources to adapt or restructure her physical, emotional, and social environment; help her consider realistic alternative plans of adaptation to life.

Betty was viewed by most of the nursing staff as a "typically good patient who never complained." She had, of course, many hospitalizations, but observation of her behavior and appearance showed evidence of tension and anxiety: her mouth was held rigidly; her almost constant smile resembled a grimace; her eyes lacked luster and were sad; and her body and arms were held rigidly. The nurse specifically designed her behavior to be such that trust could be developed; this involved listening, accepting without judgment, reflecting, using silence, making no demands, and maintaining a patient-centered interaction. Gradually, nonverbal and then verbal clues of the development of trust in the nurse emerged.

On one occasion when her creatinine, BUN, and sodium levels were high, she said, "I've been eating potato chips and a ham sandwich. Am I going to have a convulsion?" The nurse was able to clarify for Betty the rationale for her 40 gm. protein and low-sodium diet. Betty then became more relaxed and better able to adhere to her dietary regimen. When she refused to take prescribed diuretics and antihypertensives, she would exhibit changes in thought processes, mild behavior aberrations, fatigue, and depression with crying spells. An explanation of the biochemical bases for her behavior and feelings relieved a great deal of her anxiety and tension. The nurse spent increased time with Betty, encouraged her family and significant others to visit as much as possible, and involved the nursing staff in accepting her behavior and visiting her at specified intervals. Over a period of 4 weeks, her levels of serum chemistries showed an appreciable drop, she adhered to her 800 ml. fluid restriction, and her physical activity increased.

Since Betty has a scholarship to a university and is interested in mathematics, occupational therapists, family, and friends were able to stimulate her intellectually when she felt better physically. Her significant others include not only her family and peers, but two former teaching nuns. These two nuns did much for Betty's social, intellectual, psychological, and also spiritual adaptation.

At 18 years of age, Betty is sometimes a child and sometimes a woman. She expressed fears about never being married or having children, and finally about dying before she "lived." The nurse, by listening to her and collaborating with physicians, the social worker, the psychiatrist, and her significant others, presented her with alternatives and helped her to work out these fears. A strict medical regimen, maintenance hemodialysis, and a renal transplantation were discussed with her, and with help she not only expressed her feelings, but also made a list of positive and negative factors to consider in making the medical decision that would affect her future. As of now, she and her parents have decided to proceed with a renal transplantation. Her mother has been screened and accepted as the donor.

CHAPTER 14

AN ELDERLY WOMAN WITH A HYSTERECTOMY

ROSEMARY RICH

MEDICAL AND PSYCHOSOCIAL HISTORY

Mrs. MacDonald is a 75-year-old housewife who lives with her retired husband. Their two married daughters and three grandchildren live more than 500 miles away. Mrs. MacDonald is Protestant and is responsible for an adult Sunday school class. She is of Scottish and English descent. She finished high school and attended business college for 1 year.

Mrs. MacDonald has been seeing a general practitioner for several years, mainly for hypertension. Her physician prescribed reserpine and urged her to keep her weight around 135 lb. Because she has had frequent urinary infections and constipation during the last 2 years, she was referred to a gynecologist. He recommended that she be hospitalized for repair of a rectocele, cystocele, and second-degree prolapse of the uterus.

The nurse who was assigned to Mrs. MacDonald the morning after admission used McPhetridge's "Nursing History,"* to gather data about Mrs. MacDonald. The first section of this nursing history deals with patient perception and expectations related to illness and hospitalization. The nurse learned that Mrs. MacDonald came to the hospital to have her "womb removed and the walls of the birth canal fixed up." She stated that having two children had stretched her muscles. The urinary infections have been painful and a "lot of bother" because she has had to make frequent trips to the bathroom. She knows she should drink water, but forgets. She expects to be "taken to the operating room and put to sleep. I'll probably throw up afterward. That's what happened when I had my breast removed." The gynecologist has estimated that she will remain in the hospital about 2 weeks.

The most important person in Mrs. MacDonald's life is her husband. She

---

*McPhetridge, L. M.: Nursing history: One means to personalize care, Amer. J. Nurs. 68:68-75, Jan. 1968.

expects that he and his younger brother, as well as church friends, will visit often. Although Mr. MacDonald is not a very good cook, he can "make do." He has had previous experience grocery shopping, and a neighbor lady has offered to prepare his evening meals. After Mrs. MacDonald returns home, she plans to "take it easy for a few weeks." Another neighbor pops in for coffee after breakfast every morning. The MacDonald's main recreation is watching television. Mrs. MacDonald likes soap operas; her husband likes sports events; they both enjoy quiz shows.

The second section of McPhetridge's "Nursing History" deals with specific basic needs. Mrs. MacDonald related that she has had little pain since admission. She has experienced discomfort intermittently during the past 2 years. When pain was associated with voiding, she went to her physician. "He gives me some big white pills. I think he called them Gantrisin. I take two Anacin for a headache." When the nurse asked what she would like her to do to relieve pain, Mrs. MacDonald said, "Oh, you probably know more about that than I do. You'll want to give me a shot, I suppose."

Getting to sleep at night has been a problem for several years. Mrs. MacDonald said, "My doctor has me take a teaspoonful of phenobarbital. It's a red liquid. I take it with a half glass of water. It usually helps get me to sleep, but I have to get up at least once a night to go to the bathroom. I know not to take it with wine. I forgot to drink my port wine at lunch once and I took it with my phenobarb and . . . Ha! Ha! . . . I think I got drunk—at least the kitchen was spinning."

When she was asked about personal hygiene needs, Mrs. MacDonald agreed to do as much for herself as possible, but she exclaimed, "I sure wish someone would scrub my back at least once! It hasn't had a good scrubbing for years!" She has been using cold cream on her face and powder on her body. She had no preference for time of bathing: "It doesn't matter, except I can't bathe just before going to bed. It wakes me up and I can't go to sleep."

There is no tub in the MacDonald's house. Mrs. MacDonald takes a "sponge bath" at the lavatory sink, because she is afraid of falling in the shower stall. One of the daughters applied some "funny looking strips" in the shower when she visited a couple of years ago. "She didn't even ask first whether she could! How do you like that?"

Questions about safety revealed that Mrs. MacDonald had fallen several times during the last few years, and her physician recommended that she use a cane. She tried a cane for a few months. After losing two of them, she stopped because "It's more bother than it's worth."

No one has discussed staying in bed, but Mrs. MacDonald thought she would be bedfast for several days. "It's nice just to lie in bed and let other people do things for a few days." She expected to feel tired after leaving the hospital, but she also expected to manage. "I always have." She wears bifocal glasses, and her hearing is "too good, sometimes."

Mrs. MacDonald reported that the nurses are "making me drink more than usual. I know I don't drink enough, but I forget." She likes tea, root beer, and milk, especially a malted milk at bedtime. She has full dentures, but she wears them only when she goes out or when people visit. The dentures make her mouth sore. Mrs. MacDonald tends to be overweight; her physician has recommended that she "eat less, especially starchy things," to control her weight. He "scolded" her last week for being 6 pounds overweight. Her food habits have not changed because of her illness. She and her husband enjoy breakfast more than other meals. They usually have eggs, bacon, Wheaties, and whole wheat toast. Lunch is a "pick-up" of salad, cheese, and cold meat. The evening meal varies. Sometimes they eat cake and ice cream, because Mr. MacDonald is no help in planning menus and "I just run out of ideas." She encountered no problems in the hospital: "It's nice to eat someone else's cooking. I've been eating my own for—I don't know how many years—about 50, I guess."

Problems with bowel elimination have plagued Mrs. MacDonald intermittently for years. She has been using bulk-producing laxatives. She expects that the operation will eliminate the need to take laxatives. Dysuria has accompanied the bouts of bladder infection. She did not anticipate any trouble in the hospital, but she asked, "Do you think I'll have trouble?"

Mrs. MacDonald has had no problems with breathing. She was allergic to chocolate many years ago, but this does not bother her now. As the nurse started the questions about her function as a wife, Mrs. MacDonald hesitated, then said, "Say, I'm getting hoarse from all this talking. Can we stop now?"

The nurse did not know whether this remark meant that the material was difficult for Mrs. MacDonald to talk about, whether this was the wrong time to discuss her role as a wife, or whether she was tired. The nurse considered it prudent to withdraw for the time being. She said, "Of course. I'm here and I'll be in and out during the day. You know how to turn on your light, don't you?" Mrs. MacDonald answered, "Oh yes, thank you. I'll call if I want something."

PREOPERATIVE NURSING OBJECTIVES

Maintain good hygiene and physical comfort. Mrs. MacDonald had not had a "good bath" for several years. On the day before the operation, she and her nurse decided that a long, warm soaking bath would be a good idea. She splashed around for about one-half hour and enjoyed having her back scrubbed. Since her skin was very dry, superfatted soap was used; she decided she would try to find some at the grocery.

After Mrs. MacDonald's long bath, the nurse spent 40 minutes trimming her toenails. Mrs. MacDonald said she was ashamed of her feet. She soaks them once a month or so, but she cannot reach them easily. She expressed gratitude to the nurse for taking the trouble to cut her nails. The nurse asked Mrs. MacDonald whether her husband could assist her in cutting her nails. The reply was negative; so she asked whether the neighbor lady could assist her in such a task. Mrs. MacDonald stated that she had never thought about it before. She has helped her neighbor, but she would have to think about asking for help with cutting toenails.

Promote optimal activity. Although Mrs. MacDonald walked in a sprightly manner, during her bath the nurse noticed that her muscles were quite flabby. There were many varicosities on her legs.

When the history was being taken, Mrs. MacDonald said that she frequently watches TV. The nurse thought she needed more information about physical activity; so she asked about household chores. Mrs. MacDonald has adjusted to the loss of muscles which were excised at the time of the radical mastectomy. The only problem that she encounters is reaching to the top shelf of kitchen cabinets. She still does the washing and hangs it on an outside clothesline. Mr. MacDonald carries the basket to a cart that he made. It stands 3 feet off the ground and this eliminates stooping.

During the last 10 years, Mrs. MacDonald has become "a bit lax" about ironing. She said, "I just put the sheets back on the bed, and a young girl next door does the ironing—my dresses and my husband's shirts. She only charges me $2.00. That's not too much, do you think?" Mrs. MacDonald still cleans the house "once a week whether it needs it or not! It looks O.K. to me, but my younger daughter gripes about the dust everytime she visits. She doesn't know what it is to be 75 years old." Mrs. MacDonald walks three blocks to church every Sunday, but someone usually drives her home.

Information about activity and observation of Mrs. MacDonald led to a nursing diagnosis: This lady was in just fair physical condition. To help prevent postoperative complications, Mrs. MacDonald's nurse asked the physical therapist to teach postoperative leg exercises. The nurse listed the details on the nursing care plan and suggested that everyone involved remind Mrs. MacDonald to practice at least four times a day. She was informed that she would do leg exercises every hour as soon as she was awake from the anesthesia and that she would continue to do them frequently as long as she stayed in bed. Elastic stockings were ordered so that they could be applied in the recovery room.

Promote rest and sleep. Since Mrs. MacDonald often has trouble falling asleep, she was checked every half hour during the early part of the night.

Promote safety through prevention of accident. Since Mrs. MacDonald has a history of nocturia, a night light was placed so that she could see to get to the bathroom without stumbling over strange furniture. The nurse phoned Mr. MacDonald and asked him to bring her cane.

Facilitate maintenance of a supply of oxygen. Mrs. MacDonald has no history of respiratory problems. She has a forward thoracic curvature that is typical of the elderly. Another nursing diagnosis was that this lady is a likely candidate for atelectasis postoperatively. Mrs. MacDonald's nurse asked the physical therapist to teach deep breathing and segmental chest expansion. The two of them decided together that Mrs. MacDonald should practice these exercises every 3 hours preoperatively. A notation was made on the nursing care plan. The nurse predicted that IPPB would be used postoperatively; she called on the inhalation therapist to acquaint Mrs. MacDonald with the equipment. Mrs. MacDonald was apprised of the fact that she would use the IPPB machine every 4 hours for 3 or 4 days postoperatively.

Maintain nutrition. Two problems were identified: (1) Mrs. MacDonald is slightly overweight; she needs some help with a low caloric diet; (2) there is some indication that the MacDonalds are not eating balanced diets. The nurse noted these problems on the care plan. During a care conference, one member of the group reported that Mrs. MacDonald was having trouble remembering the sequence of the leg exercises. They accepted this as evidence that Mrs. MacDonald could not tolerate any more input of information at this time. A note to seek assistance from the Visiting Nurse Association (VNA) was made on the care plan. One suggestion was that the Meals-on-Wheels program in the city could provide evening meals. Being 6 lb. overweight was not thought to be a pressing problem. Mrs. MacDonald would probably lose a few pounds during the immediate postoperative period while she will be receiving I.V. fluids.

Facilitate communication about preoperative fear. During history-taking and during the tub bath, Mrs. MacDonald divulged information that served as clues that she was anxious about something. (She blurted out remarks about her family and asked the nurse questions.) That afternoon, the nurse sat in a chair by the bedside and asked whether Mrs. MacDonald would like to visit the operating and recovery rooms and whether she had any questions about the operation. Mrs. MacDonald said she did not want to use the energy to go to the recovery room, but she would appreciate another explanation of what the gynecologist planned to do. The nurse drew sketches to illustrate the procedure, and Mrs. MacDonald thanked her. As the nurse was preparing to leave, Mrs. MacDonald asked, "Do you know why they're going to give me a spinal and not put me to sleep?" This was news to the nurse; so she said she would find out. She chatted with the anesthesiologist who revealed that Mrs. MacDonald had not discontinued taking the reserpine for hypertension 2 weeks prior to admission as ordered by her physician, because she "forgot." The nurse then explained the nature of a spinal anesthetic to Mrs. MacDonald and told her that the anesthesiologist considered a spinal anesthetic to be the safest one, since she had been taking this type of medication. "Oh dear, there I go again," she added. "And while we're talking about forgetting, do you suppose someone can call Mr. MacDonald tomorrow morning at 6:30? He'll forget to set the alarm and I know he'll want to be here." A note was left for the night nurse to make this call.

Early on the day of the operation, Mr. MacDonald appeared. He accompanied Mrs. MacDonald and her nurse to the operating room and said, "I'll see you later." "O.K.," she answered. Mrs. MacDonald had a vaginal hysterectomy and anterior and posterior repair of the vaginal walls.

POSTOPERATIVE OBJECTIVES

When Mrs. MacDonald returned to her four-bed room, she expressed surprise about the spinal anesthetic. "That was much different than I thought. Certainly isn't a very dignified position, but all those sheets help a lot, don't they? I watched the whole thing in the ceiling light. I never want a general anesthetic again!" In the immediate postoperative period after she had regained function in her legs, she was reminded to do the leg exercises. The nursing staff reminded her to do these exercises when they had her cough, turn, and deep-breathe. The elastic stockings were changed, and IPPB was administered every 4 hours. Mrs. MacDonald used the IPPB reluctantly but she said that the stockings "felt good." She had a remarkably speedy recovery. Within 3 days she was telephone receptionist for the other three ladies in the room.

Maintain fluid balance. The first postoperative day, Mrs. MacDonald was maintained on I.V. fluids. The left arm was used because the radical mastectomy 30 years ago had left her right arm with limited circulation. One of the staff went to Mrs. MacDonald every hour to remind her to drink fluids. Root beer was sent from the kitchen and a milk shake was provided at night.

Maintain elimination. Mrs. MacDonald had a retention catheter for 3 days. The catheter was checked frequently to guarantee patency of the gravity bladder drainage system. On the morning of the fourth postoperative day, the catheter was removed. A urine specimen was sent for culture and sensitivity tests and a "check-void-residual" routine was begun. Three hours later, after Mrs. MacDonald had exercised by walking in the hall, the nurse helped her to the bathroom and showed her how to place a basin under the toilet seat to retain the urine for measurement. The basin was used because it allows a patient to assume a natural sitting position for voiding. Mrs. MacDonald voided 100 ml. After another exercise period in the ensuing 3 hours, Mrs. MacDonald voided again. The nursing staff checked her voiding pattern for volume and time between voidings until early evening. She was catheterized for residual after visiting hours; 60 ml. residual were obtained, and the catheterizations were discontinued. For the next 36 hours, the nurse checked Mrs. MacDonald to be certain that she was having no dysuria or bladder distention. She measured the amount to determine that Mrs. MacDonald voided at least 100 ml. each time. The nurse compared the intake-output ratio data from the previous 3 days to the ratio after the catheter was removed. She checked the frequency of voiding to help establish a 3- to 4-hour pattern of voiding.

Colace, every night, was ordered to keep stools soft. The nurse suggested to the house officer that prune juice be used in the hospital. She thought that practice in the hospital might help Mrs. MacDonald remember to use it at home. The house officer agreed that this was worth a try.

Prevent postoperative infection. Perineal irrigations with warm saline solution were used after each voiding and defecation. This procedure also provided an opportunity to discuss proper use of toilet tissue. Since urinary infections are sometimes caused by bacteria from the rectum, it is important for the nurse to stress good toilet hygiene and to teach Mrs. MacDonald to wipe herself from front to back and discard the tissue into the toilet. Mrs. MacDonald was perplexed that wiping as she had been doing might have been a cause of her bladder infection, but she said, "Now I can see how I can help not get another infection." After each irrigation an infrared lamp was used to help dry the area and promote wound healing. Mrs. MacDonald thought this was "kind of silly, but I guess you know what you're doing."

Maintain personal hygiene. The nurse assisted Mrs. MacDonald with a sponge bath the second and third postoperative days. She noted that the patient used an excessive amount of soap. Since Mrs. MacDonald would be continuing her sponge baths at home, the nurse discussed reducing the amount of soap and how to manage adequate rinsing of her skin.

On the third postoperative day, the nurse added a commercial product (such as Geri-bath) to the bath water. This preparation prevents dryness of skin, has a pleasant odor, and makes the skin feel soft and pliable. Mrs. MacDonald seemed pleased and stated that she would get the product as well as the superfatted soap.

Mrs. MacDonald asked the nurse to cut her toenails once more before she was discharged. She said, "I just can't ask my husband or neighbor to do it for me." The nurse said that she would be glad to cut her nails. "I've been thinking about how you will manage at home. Do you know about the Visiting Nurse Association?" Mrs. MacDonald replied, "Oh yes, one of the ladies down the street has a nurse come in to help her take care of her husband."

Use community resources to meet continuing needs. The nurse built upon Mrs. MacDonald's prior knowledge of the VNA to discuss ways in which a visiting nurse could help with foot care, bathing, taking medications, getting adequate rest, and planning activities of daily living. "I really would like to have a nurse come in, but I'll have to talk to my husband. He can't come today. Will you be here tomorrow?" The nurse assured her that she would be available when Mr. MacDonald visited.

The next evening, the nurse learned that the MacDonalds' greatest concern was the cost. The nurse explained that the VNA worked out with each family the assigned fee. She suggested that she ask the medical social worker to explain what assistance Medicare would provide. During the discussion, Meals-on-Wheels was mentioned. Mr. and Mrs. MacDonald thought that they would like to try having a meal sent in for one evening a week.

The days prior to discharge provided opportunity for completing transition to the home environment. The written referral to the VNA had been sent to the agency. On the day of discharge, the nurse called the VNA to discuss the referral. The visiting nurse indicated that she would see Mrs. MacDonald in 2 days.

Mrs. MacDonald's postoperative course was uncomplicated and 10 days after the day of operation, she was discharged. The nurse informed her of the anticipated date of the visiting nurse's initial visit. Mrs. MacDonald was given a card indicating an appointment in 2 weeks with her gynecologist. She understood that she could call her nurse in the hospital, if she had questions before the first VNA visit.

CHAPTER 15

CHRONIC OBSTRUCTIVE PULMONARY DISEASE AND RESPIRATORY FAILURE IN AN ELDERLY WOMAN

GAYLE TRAVER

MEDICAL HISTORY

Mrs. Nagy has chronic obstructive pulmonary disease (COPD) that was diagnosed 20 years ago. She initially denied her illness, but in recent years has acknowledged shortness of breath. In addition to COPD, Mrs. Nagy has been followed in the ambulatory care area for numerous other complaints. Her chart indicates that she has gained the reputation of being a hypochondriac.

In 1967, cor pulmonale was diagnosed as a complication of the COPD, and in August 1968, Mrs. Nagy came to the clinic complaining of increased shortness of breath. Her physician recommended that she carry out her bronchial hygiene exercises more frequently, and on her next visit the shortness of breath had decreased. Two weeks later, although her breathing continued to improve, she had developed ankle and leg edema and had gained 8 lb. Mrs. Nagy's daughter who accompanied her to the clinic stated that her mother was becoming clumsy and was dropping things. At this time, 1 ml. of Mercuhydrin was given, and Mrs. Nagy was requested to return in 1 week. At that time she had increased shortness of breath, increased edema, and a weight gain. It was also noted that she was developing senile mental changes. Although hospitalization was recommended, Mrs. Nagy refused to be admitted. Three days later, however, she returned to the clinic with an exacerbation of her symptoms. (She denied cough and sputum production.) On this visit Mrs. Nagy agreed to admission for treatment of cor pulmonale.

PSYCHOSOCIAL BACKGROUND

Mrs. Nagy is a 70-year-old Hungarian-born widow who has lived in this country for more than 40 years. Several of her children, all of whom are married, live nearby, but she lives quite independently of them. She owns her own home and lives there with her son's mother-in-law. The latter does much of the housekeeping, but Mrs. Nagy does most of her own cooking as she does not like the meals her son's mother-in-law prepares.

NURSING ASSESSMENT AND NURSING INTERVENTION

Upon admission to the floor, the nurse noted that the patient was sleepy, cyanotic, and confused. Oxygen was ordered at 2 L./min. via a nasal cannula. IPPB with air dilution for 15 minutes q.4h. and ultrasonic mist q.4h. were also ordered. The next day the nurses noted that sputum production remained scant and that the patient was more lethargic. Sometime during the morning the oxygen was increased to 5 L./min. by mistake. Mrs. Nagy became more lethargic and unable to use the IPPB apparatus. The physician, who was notified at once, discontinued the oxygen. The patient's breathing remained shallow; she was difficult to arouse; and she was still unable to use the IPPB apparatus, *even* with a face mask. The physician began to bag-breathe the patient and the anesthesiologist was called to insert an endotracheal tube. After intubation and a period of manual ventilation, arterial blood gases were drawn. The results were as follows: pO_2 33 mm. Hg (normal, 95), pCO_2 81 mm. Hg (normal, 40), pH 7.3 (normal, 7.35-7.45).

FOLLOW-UP

Mrs. Nagy's respirations were maintained by means of a respirator. Initially, a pressure-cycled machine was used, and later a volume-controlled ventilator was employed. Three days later her condition had not shown much improvement, and a tracheostomy was performed. It was not until 6 weeks later that Mrs. Nagy was finally weaned off the respirator. She eventually returned home 9 weeks after admission. In the past 2 years since this episode of acute respiratory failure, Mrs. Nagy has not required hospitalization. She has continued to live in her own home and although her activity is limited, she is still able to be relatively independent.

DISCUSSION OF NURSING CARE

This discussion concerns the nursing intervention that *should* have been initiated.

For a month before the patient was admitted, her clinical symptoms indicated decreased ventilation, her shortness of breath increased, her behavior changed, and her heart failure worsened. The knowledgeable nurse would have been alert to these changes in the patient's symptoms. It is often the nurse who has known the patient over a period of time who is aware of the subtle, gradual progression of symptoms, for a change is difficult to note if baseline observations are not readily available. Further investigation may have produced more data to substantiate the tentative diagnosis of decreased ventilation. The nurse should have also spent time with the patient and her family to be sure that they understood the importance of bronchial hygiene and understood how to carry out the treatment at home. A referral to the visiting nurse might have been very helpful.

After Mrs. Nagy was hospitalized, the nurse noted that she was confused and lethargic. Efforts should have been made to stimulate the patient at least every hour to make her deep-breathe and cough. If the patient was unable to cough productively, intratracheal suctioning may have been necessary. The nurse could also have recommended increased use of IPPB, ultrasonic mist, and the other measures used in bronchial toilet. The nurse should have closely monitored the oxygen administration to the patient, and the nurse's clinical observations should have led her to assume that Mrs. Nagy was retaining carbon dioxide even though blood gas levels were not available.

When the nurse suspects that a patient's respirations are being depressed by high levels of carbon dioxide (CO_2 narcosis), she needs to recognize that the low blood level of oxygen (pO_2) is serving as the stimulus to respiration. Thus, the amount of oxygen being administered must be closely controlled so as not to remove this hypoxic stimulus to respiration. In reviewing what happened to Mrs. Nagy, two points need emphasizing. First, IPPB with oxygen diluted with room air usually delivers more than 40% oxygen. Therefore, if there is any question that a patient is in CO_2 narcosis, it is safer to use compressed air rather than oxygen for IPPB administration. Secondly, the nasal oxygen was accidentally increased to 5 L./min. and the patient's respirations were further reduced as the hypoxic stimulus to respiration was removed. The nurse should have understood that patients with COPD are candidates for CO_2 narcosis, and therefore oxygen is usually not given at more than 1 or 2 L./min. This should be explained to all nursing personnel having contact with the patient so that no one will increase the flow rate above the prescribed level.

The patient in respiratory failure demands alert nursing observation and aggressive intervention. If such care had been available, Mrs. Nagy's condition would not have deteriorated to an apparent respiratory arrest before endotracheal intubation was performed. In fact, intubation might not have been necessary. Mrs. Nagy required intensive nursing care throughout her hospitalization. In addition to her basic physiologic need for improved ventilation, Mrs. Nagy was very depressed, frightened, and anxious. Many of the problems encountered in weaning the patient off the respirator were psychologic rather than

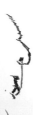

physiologic. The nurse had to motivate the patient and instill in her the will to live and the belief that she could return home. This care study has emphasized the acute physiologic needs Mrs. Nagy presented. Her other needs became increasingly evident and gained priority later in the hospitalization. Although priorities vary, all needs of a patient must be considered at all times.

CONCLUSION

The following nursing assessment outline is helpful in evaluating a patient's pulmonary condition; it includes some basic cardiovascular data that are related to pulmonary disease. A record such as this would have been useful to the staff who were taking care of Mrs. Nagy and could have been used to keep them all aware of her medical condition and psychosocial circumstances.

NURSING ASSESSMENT

IDENTIFYING INFORMATION:

Name _____ Age _____

Address _____ Sex _____

Phone _____ Circle marital status: M   S   W   D   Sep.

Diagnosis _____

_____

Reason for referral _____

_____

Referral from _____

Patient's chief complaint _____

Medical orders _____   _____

_____   _____

_____   _____

Continued.

NURSING ASSESSMENT—cont'd

BACKGROUND INFORMATION:

Occupation _____

Cultural group _____

Living arrangements: Dwelling _____

Family members _____

Awareness and understanding of illness _____

_____

_____

Family understanding and support _____

_____

_____

Interests and socialization _____

_____

	Yes	No
PULMONARY HISTORY:		
Short of breath?		
If yes, duration: _____		
If yes, at rest?		
with activities of daily living (ADL)?		
with ambulation?		
with exercise?		
Cough?		
If yes, duration: _____		

NURSING ASSESSMENT—cont'd

PULMONARY HISTORY: Yes | No

Sputum production? ....

If yes, volume per day: _____

Description: Consistency _____

Color_____

If recent change in sputum production, describe: _____

Does patient do respiratory therapy at home? ....

IPPB ....

Hand nebulizer ....

Mist ....

O_2 (continuous, intermittent) ....

Postural drainage ....

Has patient been under medical and/or nursing supervision? ....

PHN (VNA) _____ OPD _____ Private physician _____

PRESENT STATUS:

Pulmonary

Respiratory rate _____ Depth (tidal volume) _____

Is pattern regular? ....

irregular in depth? ....

in rate? ....

Is chest movement symmetrical? ....

Is pattern thoracic? _____ Diaphragmatic? _____

Continued.

NURSING ASSESSMENT—cont'd

PRESENT STATUS:

Pulmonary   Yes | No

Are accessory muscles used? ...._____|_____

Is nasal flaring present? ...._____|_____

Is retraction present? ...._____|_____

     If yes, intercostal? _____   Substernal? _____

Is expiration prolonged? ...._____|_____

     If yes, associated with wheezing? ...._____|_____

         associated with pursed-lip breathing? ...._____|_____

Is patient dyspneic? ...._____|_____

     If yes, at rest? ...._____|_____

         with activities of daily living? ...._____|_____

         with ambulation? ...._____|_____

         with exercise? ...._____|_____

Is speech in short, clipped phrases? ...._____|_____

Is cough present? ...._____|_____

     If yes, productive of sputum? ...._____|_____

         If yes, volume per day: _____

         Description of sputum: consistency _____

                     color _____

     Is there a recent change in volume and/or color? ....|_____|_____

   Is suction necessary? ...._____|_____

NURSING ASSESSMENT—cont'd

PRESENT STATUS:

Pulmonary   Yes | No

Is chest pain present? ....

If yes, location: _____

Description: sharp _____   dull _____

constant _____   intermittent _____

Is pain induced by activity? ....

by deep breathing? ....

Is pain relieved by position? ....

medication? ....

other? _____

Cardiovascular

Heart rate _____ regular? ....

irregular in rate? ....

in volume? ....

Blood pressure _____

Does patient complain of: orthopnea? ....

paroxysmal nocturnal dyspnea (PND)? ...

Is there venous distension such as in neck veins? ....

Is there peripheral edema? ....

If yes, to what level? _____

Is it pitting? ....

Is it position dependent? ....

Has there been a recent weight gain unrelated to dietary intake? .....

Continued.

NURSING ASSESSMENT—cont'd

PRESENT STATUS: Yes | No

Skin

    Turgor: good _____   poor _____

    Color: flushed _____   cyanotic _____

Mental status

    State of consciousness: alert _____   somnolent _____

        stuporous _____ semicomatose _____ comatose _____

    Memory: recent? ...._____ | _____

             remote? ...._____ | _____

    Orientation: person? ...._____ | _____

             place? ...._____ | _____

             time? ...._____ | _____

    Follows instructions: simple? ...._____ | _____

             complex? ...._____ | _____

             variable? ...._____ | _____

Behavior:

    anxious _____   hyperactive _____

    demanding _____   hostile _____

    depressed _____   hypoactive _____

    restless _____   irritable _____

    fearful _____   short attention span _____

Has patients' mental status and behavior changed recently? ...._____ | _____

CHAPTER 16

A MAN IN ACUTE RESPIRATORY FAILURE

ELAINE NICHOLS

OBJECTIVES OF THIS STUDY

To discuss the medical care and nursing responsibilities of a patient with pneumonia superimposed on residual effects from polio.

To illustrate a nursing staff's reactions to a "demanding" patient and to suggest possible approaches to improve the nurse-patient relationship.

MEDICAL AND PSYCHOSOCIAL BACKGROUND

Mr. Bruce Johnson is a 60-year-old married retired executive whose family consists of his wife, a son, and three daughters. In 1953, at the age of 43 while vacationing in New England, Mr. Johnson developed the symptoms of a cold—malaise, fever, rhinitis, and aching joints. After returning home, he developed weakness in his legs and by the time he presented himself at the emergency room of a large university hospital, the weakness had involved his arms, and he was having difficulty breathing. The diagnosis was anterior poliomyelitis. Mr. Johnson spent the next 10 months at the hospital in a tank respirator. The residual effects of the polio were moderately weakened leg muscles, minimal to absent motor function in the right arm and hand, moderate motor activity of the left forearm and hand, and moderate weakness of the intercostal and diaphragmatic muscles.

Upon discharge from the hospital, Mr. Johnson went to a rehabilitation center for muscle-strengthening exercises of his arms and legs. He refused to learn activities of daily living (ADL) during his rehabilitation program and gave as the reason that he could not possibly "exert the energy that it would take to learn activities of daily living such as feeding, bathing, and dressing. I would rather pay someone to do those things for me so that I have the energy to go to work." As a result of this attitude and the fact that he did have sufficient money to have the ADL done for him, he relied on male attendants and family members to bathe and dress him and assist him during ambulation.

During the 17 years that elapsed between the initial bout with polio and this hospital admission, Mr. Johnson remained physically stable. He relied on a cuirass ventilator during the night to assist his weakened respiratory muscles. The cuirass ventilator fits around the anterior chest and abdomen and produces inspiration by creating a vacuum around the anterior chest and abdomen, thereby actually sucking air into the lungs and then allowing passive expiration to follow.[3] His physical care was provided by male attendants who spent long hours at his home and office. He structured his day and his care to conserve energy: he arose at a certain time each morning, was assisted with showering and dressing, leaned against a counter to eat meals, rode in a wheelchair to the car, and was driven to work. Despite the physical disability, Mr. Johnson managed his own business until 1968. He kept a second cuirass ventilator at work in case he felt the need for respiratory assistance during the day. In 1968, he sold his business and became chairman of the board of a large corporation. He managed most of the duties of chairman from his home where he had head-set phones installed in every room of the house so that he could communicate with members of the board at any time.

It was apparent from the preceding information that the patient maintained control and consistency over his disability by providing himself with the assistance he deemed necessary—manpower as well as machines—and that he maintained productivity through his work. These concepts of control, assistance (dependency), productivity, and consistency came to play a very important part during his present hospital stay. Three days prior to admission, Mr. Johnson developed an upper respiratory tract infection (URI). The development of a URI in a person with preexisting respiratory pathology is a very real crisis. In the words of Mrs. Johnson, "We have dreaded this for 17 years."

Mr. Johnson's preexisting respiratory pathology was classified as a restrictive ventilatory defect. Restrictive ventilatory defects are caused by skeletal deformities of the chest wall or thoracic spine, or by dysfunction of the intercostal and other thoracic muscles as was the case with Mr. Johnson. This restrictive defect results in a low vital capacity. Superimposed on this restrictive defect was the URI that produced obstructive disease and diffusion problems—obstructive in the sense of blockage of airways by secretions and oxygen diffusion problems across the alveolar-capillary membrane caused by inflammatory changes in the membrane.[3]

HOSPITALIZATION SUMMARY

The time span of this study encompasses a 4½-week period from the day of admission to the day of discharge from the pulmonary intensive care unit (PICU) to a general medical-surgical unit. This summary is an attempt to give the medical treatment, the nursing responsibilities, and the appearance of patient and nursing problems in chronologic order.

First week

Mr. Johnson was initially admitted to a private medical-surgical unit in fair condition. He brought with him his cuirass ventilator, a heating pad, his own roll of sheepskin, a wheelchair, and his male attendants. The diagnosis of pulmonary insufficiency caused by pneumonia in the left lung was made by chest x-ray and physical examination. The initial therapy consisted of antibiotics and rest, but Mr. Johnson's condition did not improve. When it became obvious that more aggressive therapy was necessary, he was transferred to the PICU. In the PICU, orders were written to begin vigorous pulmonary toilet; monitoring of vital signs and blood gases; intake and output; and frequent checking of skin color, state of consciousness, and amount, color, and consistency of sputum. Tetracycline, 600 mg., was ordered to be given every 6 hours to chemically combat the pneumonia. Pulmonary toilet consisted of ultrasonic mist therapy, intermittent positive pressure breathing (IPPB), postural drainage with clapping and vibrating, and deep tracheobronchial suctioning.

IPPB was administered by a pressure-cycled ventilator, the PR-1, and was given every hour for 15 minutes. Pressure-cycled ventilators are regulated by a preset pressure; the inspiratory cycle continues until a predetermined pressure is reached, the machine then turns off, and the expiratory cycle begins. Preceding each positive pressure treatment, ultrasonic mist therapy was given for 15 minutes. The purpose of this treatment was to deliver water in the form of a very fine mist deep into the lungs in order to liquefy secretions. Once secretions are liquefied, the positive pressure treatment serves to move the secretions upward to a point where they can be coughed out by the patient. In Mr. Johnson's case, however, effective coughing was impossible because of the weakness of his respiratory muscles. For this reason, deep tracheobronchial suctioning was instituted after IPPB therapy and at other times as necessary.

In addition to the intensive pulmonary toilet, careful intake and output records were kept. The recording of intake includes not only oral and intravenous fluids, but water from the ultrasonic mist treatments. A patient receiving continuous ultrasonic nebulization can receive more than 1 L. of water in a 24-hour period.[6] Urinary output, along with blood pressure and pulse, is used as an indicator of the effect of positive pressure therapy upon the circulatory system. During normal, unassisted breathing, the downward motion of the diaphragm creates negative pressure within the chest cavity. This negative pressure not only facilitates air entry into the lungs, but also facilitates blood movement from the vena cava into the right heart. During assisted ventilation, positive pressure is used to force air into the lungs during inspiration. This positive pressure may enhance air flow but can impede movement of blood from the vena cava to the heart. Therefore, under conditions necessitating high positive pressures to move air into the lungs, the heart may not receive adequate blood supply. The end result is decreased cardiac output manifesting itself through such signs as increasing pulse, decreasing blood pressure, and decreasing urinary output.[2]

Blood gas studies were instituted to assess the adequacy of ventilation and pulmonary toilet. Blood is obtained from either the brachial or femoral artery and analyzed for pH (normal, 7.35 to 7.45), pO_2 (normal, 95 to 100 mm. Hg), pCO_2 (normal, 40 mm. Hg), and O_2 saturation (normal, 90% to 96%).

The oxygen tension (pO_2) reflects the amount of oxygen that has diffused across the alveolar-capillary membrane into the arterial blood. The carbon dioxide tension (pCO_2) reflects changes in the amount of circulating carbonic acid; therefore, an elevated pCO_2 is an indication of increased amounts of carbonic acid, which results when there is a decreased ability of the lungs to excrete CO_2. The pH reflects changes in the acid-base balance of the blood. In respiratory situations, pH reflects the balance between carbonic acid and bicarbonate, which normally exists in a ratio of 1:20. In some cases, pCO_2 can be seen to directly affect pH, in that increasing pCO_2 causes increasing levels of carbonic acid and increasing levels of acid causes a drop in pH. In other instances, blood gas studies of patients with chronic obstructive pulmonary disease may not demonstrate this cause and effect relationship. Oxygen saturation reflects the amount of oxygen that will combine with hemoglobin at a given oxygen tension.

Another measure of adequate ventilation is the measuring of tidal volume (TV), vital capacity (VC), and minute tidal volume (MV). Tidal volume represents the volume of air in a single normal inhalation and exhalation. Normal values are between 500 and 600 ml. Vital capacity represents the volume of air in a single deep inhalation followed by a forced exhalation. Normal values are approximately 4800 ml. for males and 3200 ml. for females. Minute tidal volume represents the volume of air that is moved into and out of the lungs during normal respiration for 1 minute. Minute tidal volume can be determined by multiplying the respiratory rate for 1 minute by the tidal volume. On admission to the PICU, Mr. Johnson's TV was less than 150 ml., and his vital capacity was about 800 ml. This accurately reflects his restrictive plus obstructive lung defects. These parameters of ventilation (TV, VC, and MV) are measured while the patient is both on and off the ventilator. In this particular case, the nursing staff had to note also which ventilator was being used. For example, 10:00 A.M.: TV-100 ml. off; 400 ml. on PR-1.

In between treatments Mr. Johnson used his cuirass ventilator continually. He felt that he was too tired to attempt breathing on his own. He gave verbal directions to all nursing staff who cared for him on the application of his cuirass. His directions also carried over into areas such as the time for breakfast, the time for morning care, the time for pulmonary toilet, the time and how to get him out of bed and into his wheelchair, and how to position him while in bed. Because of the weakness in both arms, he needed to be fed, and he also needed secretions wiped from his mouth.

On the fourth day of his stay, it was becoming increasingly apparent that the pulmonary toilet and suctioning were not effective. The pO_2 remained low and chest X-ray films showed increasing infiltration in the left lower lobe. It was also apparent by the fourth day that Mr. Johnson was becoming weaker. He could no longer breathe deeply enough to cycle the PR-1 ventilator, and his tidal volumes were averaging below 100 ml. A cuffed endotracheal tube was inserted and a PR-2, an automatic-cycling pressure ventilator, was substituted for the PR-1. At this time he was transferred to a rocking bed. The purpose of the rocking bed was to utilize the pressure of the abdominal contents against the diaphragm as an aid during respiration. Deep tracheal suctioning was more effective through the endotracheal tube, and large amounts of thick yellow-green sputum were obtained. However, bronchial suctioning was difficult because of the acute angle of the left main stem bronchus from the trachea, which creates more difficulty in entering the left bronchus with a suction catheter than in entering the right main stem bronchus. Intravenous fluids were also started to ensure that adequate fluid intake was maintained. In Mr. Johnson's case, adequate fluid intake was especially important because an adequate circulating fluid volume serves to maintain the moistness of the mucous lining of the respiratory tract, thereby keeping secretions liquefied.

After he was intubated, Mr. Johnson could not speak, and because of his weak hands, he could not write. There were many things that he needed to communicate; so he began making clicking noises with his lips and teeth to signal that he needed attention. He also banged on the bed, or the side of the ventilator with his left arm. When the nurses approached his bed, Mr. Johnson would mouth words, and the staff would attempt to read his lips to interpret what he needed. This was very frustrating for both Mr. Johnson and the nursing staff.

Three days after intubation, the process in the left lung remained unchanged. A tracheostomy was performed because of the policy that an endotracheal tube should not be used for more than 48 hours.

Second week

Mr. Johnson was taken off the rocking bed after 3 days because of nausea and personal request. He was returned to a hospital bed for 1 day, and then the medical staff decided to put him on a CircOlectric bed so that turning to various positions could be easier and more frequent, and with the hope that frequent turning would increase the drainage from the left lower lobe. With the change to the CircOlectric bed came a change in respirators from the PR-2 to the MA-1, a volume-cycled respirator. Volume-cycled ventilators are regulated by a preset volume of air that is to be delivered to the lungs during inspiration. The inspiratory cycle of the ventilator continues until the predetermined volume of air is delivered to the lungs, then the machine shuts off, and the expiratory cycle begins. Now came 2 days of rigid turning schedule from the position of Trendelenberg, to reverse Trendelenberg, to supine, and to prone. The pulmonary toilet was maintained along with care of the tracheostomy and the monitoring of the volumes of air being delivered to the lungs by the MA-1. The suctioning was removing more and more secretions, and the pO_2 finally began to rise from 56 to 82 mm. Hg.

During all these changes, Mr. Johnson was extremely apprehensive and agitated. He expressed his feelings by more frequent and louder sounds with his lips and teeth and increased banging on the respirator. After 2 days on the CircOlectric bed, he was moved back to his own bed. With the noticeable improvement in his blood gases, the medical staff decided to begin using the cuirass ventilator instead of the MA-1. The "weaning" process from the MA-1 to the cuirass was very traumatic for medical staff, nursing staff, and Mr. Johnson. The regimen for such weaning must be planned to encompass several days. Some patients will progress faster than others, but in most instances, weaning is not accomplished within a few hours. The length of time that the weaning process will take for any one patient can be estimated if several questions are explored: How long has the patient been on the respirator from which he is being weaned? How similar to the respirator that the patient is using is the breathing aid to which he is being weaned? To what degree is the patient emotionally and physiologically dependent on his present respirator?

The weaning process was not tolerated well at all by Mr. Johnson. His needs for his mouth to be wiped and for other assistance increased during the time he was on the cuirass, and his TV on the cuirass was only between 75 ml. and 100 ml. After 24 hours of attempted weaning, Mr. Johnson was put back on the MA-1 ventilator.

The second week, like the first week, was characterized by many changes in the medical treatment. Mr. Johnson's apprehension bordered on panic during many of the changes, and by the end of the second week, he was mentally and physically exhausted. One new problem that emerged during the second week was the nursing staff's attitude toward Mr. Johnson. They were becoming increasingly frustrated by their inability to communicate with him and increasingly irritated by his lip-smacking and respirator-pounding. This behavior was increased twofold during the night, and it was from the night staff that comments first began to be heard such as "I can't stand to take care of him," or "He's the type of patient that once I am through taking care of him, I avoid seeing him again," or "I get so angry with him!"

Third week

The third week was characterized by a rigorous schedule of weaning from the MA-1 to the cuirass. Nasal O_2 at 4 L./min. was given to Mr. Johnson while he was on the cuirass and this seemed to facilitate the weaning process. At the end of the third week, the tracheostomy tube was removed and Mr. Johnson regained his voice.

The attitude of the nursing staff toward the patient was becoming worse. He was labeled as "demanding" and the nursing staff was still feeling very frustrated in attempting to meet his needs. (This problem reached its peak before Mr. Johnson regained his voice.) The nursing staff realized during the third week that this was a problem with which they needed some help. The intervention they chose was a group conference with a psychiatric nurse clinician. This group conference gave them a chance to sit down and talk about their feelings toward this patient—to actually come out and say that they really felt angry, hostile, irritated, and frustrated. Once these feelings were expressed, the clinician began exploring ways in which the situation could be alleviated. The following suggestions were given by the psychiatric nurse clinician during the conference with the nursing staff in dealing with Mr. Johnson:

1. Attempt to decipher what it is the patient is actually "demanding." In Mr. Johnson's case, the nursing staff decided that he was frightened when he thought they were not watching him; so he would call them just to have someone close by. He was also testing the staff for someone he could trust by having them do many things for him. When, instead, the staff avoided him, he could not develop this trust, and the demanding continued. Trust, confidence, and consistency could have been provided for Mr. Johnson by assigning the same people to care for him.

2. The staff was irritated by his methods of communicating when he could not speak and by his demanding behavior. Modifying these "demanding" behaviors was also a necessary approach in the improvement of the nurse-patient

relationship in this case. The following were suggestions for modifying the demanding behavior:

    a. Feed back the patient's nonverbal communication to tell him that his messages are being received.

    b. Provide another method of communicating, such as a small bell hung on the side rail.

    c. Note when the patient calls the nurse to his bedside. The staff stated that as soon as they would get to the nurses' station, he would be calling them back. Suggestions by the clinician for modifying this behavior were:

        (1) Before leaving his bedside, ask him if there is anything more that can be done for him.

        (2) Take a few steps from the bedside, turn around and return to him, and again ask if there is anything the nurse can do for him.

        (3) Tell him exactly how much time is available for him each time the nurse is giving him care and assure him of the nurse's return after other duties.

        (4) If there is no work in the nurses' station at a particular time, sit at his bedside rather than at the station.

During the group conference with the clinician, several things became apparent. Each staff member had collected information about the patient, but had not shared it with her co-workers. The feelings of frustration had been present in some of the staff members for a long period of time, but each person hesitated to state his feelings. Even when problems of nurse-patient interaction became known, the staff as a group hesitated to seek intervention. By the time the conference was held, the problems no longer existed, and even though the conference provided a "ventilation" session for the staff, approaches suggested by the clinician could not be implemented.

Fourth week

With the return of Mr. Johnson's voice, everyone's frustrations decreased significantly. By this time the nursing staff was used to Mr. Johnson's preferences, and Mr. Johnson was accustomed to the ways in which the staff did things for him, so that his requests diminished greatly. He was breathing on his own, he was able to sit in his wheelchair for increasing periods of time, and he had his wife bring in some "talking books" to listen to. On the day of discharge from the PICU, his blood gases without supplemental oxygen were pH 7.43; pO_2 70.6 mm. Hg; pCO_2 41 mm. Hg; TV 400 ml.; VC 1000 ml.; and MV 8 L.

REFERENCES

1. Comroe, J.: Physiology of respiration, Chicago, 1965, Year Book Medical Publishers, Inc.
2. Heironimus, T.: Mechanical artificial ventilation, Springfield, Ill., 1967, Charles C Thomas, Publisher.
3. Myers, J.: An orientation to chronic disease and disability, New York, 1965, The Macmillan Co.
4. Robinson, L.: Psychological aspects of the care of hospitalized patients, Philadelphia, 1968, F. A. Davis Co.
5. Schoen, E.: Clinical problem: the demanding, complaining patient, Nurs. Clin. N. Amer. 2:715-724, Dec. 1967.
6. Secor, J.: Patient care in respiratory problems, Philadelphia, 1969, W. B. Saunders Co.

CHAPTER 17

POSTOPERATIVE CARE OF A WOMAN WITH A COLOSTOMY

MARILYN J. HOWE

MEDICAL HISTORY

Mrs. Lincoln presented herself at the hospital because of vaginal bleeding. Physical examination revealed a mass in her lower left quadrant. A routine "tumor work-up" (X-rays, sigmoidoscopy, cystoscopy, and blood tests) supported the initial diagnosis—carcinoma of the ovary that involved the posterior aspect of the pelvis, including the sigmoid colon.

She had a total abdominal hysterectomy, a bilateral salpingo-oophorectomy, a partial resection of the sigmoid colon, an omentectomy, establishment of a colostomy of the descending colon, and establishment of a mucoid fistula from the proximal end of the rectum to the skin in the lower abdomen (midline).

PSYCHOSOCIAL BACKGROUND

Mrs. Lincoln is a 70-year-old widow whose husband died 20 years ago. Her two married daughters live in the city, and they both bring their families to visit and help their mother with grocery shopping. Mrs. Lincoln lives alone on the first floor of a duplex building. She enjoys working in her small garden during summers and keeps plants in her home. She likes to read the newspaper and magazines, such as *Look* and *Life*. Mrs. Lincoln does not attend church regularly, but listens to church services on the radio and reads her Bible. The neighbors from the second floor visit her occasionally.

LABORATORY DATA

All laboratory work was within normal limits upon admission. Hematocrit fell from 42 to 33 vol.% within 24 hours postoperatively (normal, 37 to 47 vol.%).

NURSING CARE OBJECTIVES

Maintain skin integrity; prevent infection of wound and skin around retention sutures; provide control of products of bowel elimination. On the third postoperative day, after removal of the initial dressings, a temporary colostomy appliance was applied. An open-ended appliance was chosen to reduce the necessity of changing the adhesive-backed appliance frequently. The open end allowed for cleaning the inside of the bag without removal of the appliance. Clinically, skin integrity may be effectively maintained if a 24-hour seal can be achieved.

Mrs. Lincoln's skin was cleaned with soap and water, rinsed, and then dried. A skin test revealed no allergy to tincture of benzoin. The skin to be covered by the adhesive backing of the appliance was painted with a layer of tincture of benzoin. The benzoin was allowed to dry until tacky and karaya gum powder was sprinkled over the area. The excess karaya was dusted off and another layer of tincture of benzoin applied. When this layer was tacky to touch, the appliance was pressed firmly onto the skin.

On the fifth postoperative day, copious liquid stools began to discharge from the colostomy. A karaya gum seal was placed around the appliance stoma opening to prevent leakage of the liquid stool. The skin preparation, use of the karaya seal, and temporary appliance regimen were continued for 10 days.

Help Mrs. Lincoln assume responsibility for her own care:

Take care to speak in an objective fashion.

Describe steps for skin care and for application of the appliance.

Get her involved: ask whether she wants to know about skin care and whether she wants to look at her stoma.

Mrs. Lincoln was slow in becoming involved. She would not look at the colostomy, and when she was asked whether she wanted to know about skin care, she said, "I don't think I *can* learn." Finally, she agreed to "try" when asked whether she would make step-by-step efforts. She began to ask questions such as, "Will you make sure I know before I go home? Will you see that I don't hurt myself?"

The approach used with Mrs. Lincoln was to cast her into the role of student. It was thought important to convey to her that making a mistake was not tragic and to also convey confidence in her ability to learn to care for herself. She was encouraged to ask questions and to express herself openly and honestly.

Assess Mrs. Lincoln as a learner. In the 10-day period prior to being fitted with a permament appliance, Mrs. Lincoln was increasingly able to ambulate for greater distances and to stay out of bed for longer periods. She was eating solid foods and was started on an oral iron preparation.

Mrs. Lincoln displayed her self-management by insisting to "do things for myself." She could do most of her bathing with the exception of her back and feet. She kept her section of a semiprivate room organized and made it known that "everything has its place." She talked about her household plants and related that no one could look after them as well as she could. Her oldest daughter was taking care of the plants and her home, but Mrs. Lincoln never seemed satisfied with her daughter's report on the home management. Mrs. Lincoln described what fine daughters she has and said that they have often insisted that she come live with them. However, she likes her home and the independence she has there where she can do as she pleases.

Although Mrs. Lincoln has arthritis, she seemed to have adequate motor function in her hands. She broke her glasses 10 years ago, but never bothered to have them replaced. She apparently has some myopia, but when she held her Bible or the newspaper close to her face, she could manage to read.

Mrs. Lincoln appeared socially astute and could carry on a conversation with the nursing staff or her roommates; the conversation was usually punctuated with long silences. She did not appear to have any marked hearing deficit. She could express feelings of impatience when the nursing staff did not get things done when she wanted them done. She could join in with the staff as they enjoyed chatting with patients, and she joined in the staffs' organized coffee klatsches.

Her conversation seemed to indicate that Mrs. Lincoln was afraid she was too old to learn, but once she understood and could do a task she was not very forgetful. She was offered opportunities to learn skin care, to apply the appliance, and to manage colostomy irrigations step-by-step and with sufficient practice. The practice sessions would continue until she thought she could manage at home. She appeared to think the proposed teaching plan would be suitable, provided that she had supervision, so that she "wouldn't do anything wrong."

Implement the teaching plan. Fifteen days after surgery Mrs. Lincoln was fitted with a permanent colostomy appliance. The appliance had a lightweight flexible plastic face-plate. The adjustable elastic belt had a snap-lock jaw arrangement for holding the face-plate and the disposable bags together as a unit. This simple appliance was devised specifically for persons who have arthritis affecting their fingers. The flexible plastic face-plate tends to remain in place better than, for example, metal face-plates, This permanent appliance is matched by an irrigating set for which the same face-plate and disposable irrigating plastic bags are used. The irrigating bags are long enough to reach into the toilet bowl and attach to the face-plate in the same manner as the single-service colostomy pouches.

Mrs. Lincoln's stools were, by this time, semisolid, and she seemed able to visualize her stoma clearly enough to center the face-plate. On the evening of the fourteenth postoperative day, the nurse demonstrated the appliance and named each of the pieces. Mrs. Lincoln watched the demonstration and then returned the demonstration by putting the appliance together. Her assignment for the remainder of the evening was to put the appliance together at least four more times. On the next day she was expected to wear the permanent appliance. She was also to do her own skin care and change the single-service pouches when necessary. She was assured that each time she took care of her colostomy, she would have supervision.

By this time, Mrs. Lincoln had touched her stoma. She had progressed from referring to her colostomy as "it" or the "thing" to using "my stoma" or "my colostomy." The nursing staff had been careful during these 2 weeks to use "your colostomy" or "your stoma," but not to push Mrs. Lincoln into using personalized terminology.

During the fifteenth postoperative day, Mrs. Lincoln with minimal assistance, managed cleaning her skin with soap and water and then drying the skin. She was able to put the appliance together and center the face-plate. She had to change the single-service pouches four times and managed this task without much difficulty. She seemed pleased with herself and commented, "Now I know I can do it. Before, I thought I would have to stay at home all the time. I think I can go to church if I feel up to it." When asked if she was ready to learn colostomy irrigation, she looked at the nurse sideways, grinned, and then replied, "Whenever you are ready."

That evening, Mrs. Lincoln was shown how to do her colostomy irrigation. The plan was for the nurse to do the irrigation the first time and to have Mrs. Lincoln return the demonstration the next evening. Each of the steps of the irrigation was explained, and she was involved to the extent of holding the tubing and the backflow disk, putting on the face-plate and elastic belt, and adjusting the irrigating bags.

After the irrigation, the nurse and Mrs. Lincoln reviewed the steps. While Mrs. Lincoln described the procedure, the nurse wrote the steps in the patient's language on 5 × 8 inch cards in large print. The cards could serve as reminders to Mrs. Lincoln after her return home. She indicated that Hazel, her oldest daughter, would come in the next evening and learn how to do the procedure.

Mrs. Lincoln was concerned about the odor from her colostomy as well as the odor from the mucoid fistula. She was given deodorant tablets to crush and place in the single-service colostomy pouch. For her, these tablets seemed to be effective. She washed the mucoid fistula opening with soap and water and covered the area with a 4 × 4 inch gauze pad that had been folded over and taped in place. One drop of oil of peppermint on the 4 × 4 inch pad seemed effective in controlling the odor.

The nurse and Mrs. Lincoln had spent several sessions talking about her diet management. A special low-residue, low–gas forming food list had been obtained. She was able to think back about foods that seemed to produce gas and foods that either constipated her or gave her diarrhea previously. She thought the list would be a good reference and stated that she could manage her dietary needs. The discussion was also focused on foods high in iron content and included ways to provide sufficient protein in her diet.

On the evening of the sixteenth postoperative day, Mrs. Lincoln's oldest daughter participated in the colostomy irrigations. Mrs. Lincoln provided the directions, while she and her daughter managed the procedure. Mrs. Lincoln had several steps mixed up, but demonstrated what the nurse thought to be remarkable recall as well as apparent ease in handling the equipment. She did not appear to be uneasy about doing digital dilatation of her stoma and insisted that her daughter learn how to dilate the stoma. After an initial period of discomfort, her daughter appeared to manage equally as well as Mrs. Lincoln and the two of them seemed to be an effective team.

The nurse complimented Mrs. Lincoln on being such a fast learner. Her reply was that once she understood what needed to be done, she just "got down to learning it. Last night," she continued, "I just went over the steps in my mind until I got it. You can give our list to Hazel—she might need it."

Mrs. Lincoln's daughter seemed pleased when she, too, was complimented on her skill. She stated, "When Mama told me that she wanted my help, I was glad I could do it. The doctor wants her to stay with me for 2 weeks before she goes to her own place."

This last statement started an argument that continued into the next day when Hazel returned. The physician joined Hazel, and in the end Mrs. Lincoln agreed to the 2-week period, "but not a minute longer." When the physician asked Mrs. Lincoln when she would be ready to go home, she answered that she would go as soon as she and her daughter did one more irrigation. The nurse was to observe and see that they did everything right. All their home-going supplies were ready. The nurse had written on cards the skin care procedure; the procedure for modifying the permanent colostomy bag if Mrs. Lincoln should develop diarrhea (she was scheduled for radiation therapy in 2 weeks); the irrigation procedure; and a card with the nurse's phone numbers and several places where she could obtain supplies.

Mrs. Lincoln continued the account of how she would manage her diet and how much exercise she would get each day. She agreed she would call the nurse if she had difficulty with any of her activities of daily living, such as bathing or elimination. She had been consulted about having a visiting nurse, but she and her daughter really did not need any assistance. She would be back at the clinic in 1 week and expected the physician to see to it that she obtained an appointment in the eye clinic so that she could get some glasses. The physician agreed that she was ready for transition to her home environment and he planned to see her in a week and to arrange for the eye clinic appointment.

Both mother and daughter demonstrated their competence for colostomy irrigation, got everything together, and were on their way home in 2 hours. The nurse shared with the nursing personnel in the clinic Mrs. Lincoln's ability to determine and to use human and material resources, as well as her ability to evaluate her own progress. The remainder of her nursing care plan (not included in this care study) was also shared with the nursing personnel.

CHAPTER 18

NURSING REQUIREMENTS OF A WOMAN
WITH A CHOLECYSTECTOMY

ROXIE FERNELIUS

MEDICAL HISTORY

Mrs. Laura Summers, age 45, is a white woman who was admitted to the hospital for removal of her gallbladder. She has had recurrent attacks of right upper quadrant pain with some nausea and vomiting, especially after eating, over the past several months. The diagnosis of chronic cholecystitis with cholelithiasis was made on the basis of X-ray studies in which a stone was visualized in the gallbladder. Her medical history was essentially negative.

PSYCHOSOCIAL BACKGROUND

Mrs. Summers, a housewife, is a slightly obese woman with brown hair who likes to bake and sew and has also been somewhat active in school and church activities. Her husband is a successful salesman in a furniture store where he has Blue Cross insurance coverage. The couple has two teen-age children, and the family lives in the city where they are buying their own home. Mrs. Summers speaks proudly of her children who are keeping house while she is hospitalized. Her husband visits daily, and both he and the children are supportive and concerned. They have sent flowers and cards.

LABORATORY RESULTS

All laboratory findings were negative except the direct bilirubin, which was 2 mg./100 ml. (normal, 0.1 to 1.2).

NURSING INTERVENTION—PREOPERATIVE PHASE

Mrs. Summers was admitted to the hospital early on Sunday afternoon for surgery Monday morning. When the nurse admitted Mrs. Summers to her private room, she learned that the patient had never been in the hospital except for the birth of her two children. Mrs. Summers seemed anxious to learn about what would happen to her in the next few hours. After routine blood and urine specimens were obtained, she was allowed to visit with her husband who was told that he could come to see her at 7:00 A.M. the next morning before she went to surgery.

The admitting nurse drew up the following plan for Mrs. Summers' preoperative care that evening:

OBJECTIVES	APPROACH
Assess what Mrs. Summers knows about the impending surgery.	Determine what the doctor has told her. Ask her if she has any questions. Draw a diagram of the incision and T-tube if indicated. Allow her to express any fears.
Review postoperative care.	Will go to the recovery room from the operating room and remain there until she is awake. Will have a nasogastric tube in her nose connected to suction to prevent abdominal distention. Will have a T-tube coming out of her incision that will drain bile into a bottle; her dressing will be changed as necessary. Will receive I.V. fluids for 1 or 2 postoperative days. Will be asked to turn, cough, and deep-breathe often after surgery, and she will be up out of bed the day after surgery. All of these will be done to help her recover as rapidly as possible and without complications.
Prepare her for surgery.	Explain the need for the preoperative shave and enema and carry out these procedures. Have her take a shower with a hexachlorophene soap. Administer sleeping medication (secobarbital, 100 mg.). Remove pitcher from room and explain that she is to have nothing orally after midnight. Explain that she will be awakened in the morning so that she can void, wash her hands and face, and brush her teeth. She will then be dressed in a hospital gown and cap and will be given a preanesthetic hypodermic. Her husband may remain with her until she is taken to surgery.

SURGERY

A cholecystectomy with common bile duct exploration and T-tube insertion was performed under general anesthesia. Mrs. Summers received 1500 ml. of 5% glucose in saline during surgery. She was taken to the recovery room in good condition.

POSTOPERATIVE ORDERS

June 2 Vital signs q.15min. until stable.

Keep I.V. tubing open with 1000 ml. of 5% glucose in water.

Levin tube to low suction.

Irrigate Levin tube with 20 ml. of normal saline p.r.n.

Meperidine HCl (Demerol), 100 mg., q.3-4h. p.r.n. for pain.

June 3 Keep I.V. tubing open, alternating 1000 ml. of 5% glucose in water with 1000 ml. of 5% glucose in saline.

Discontinue Levin tube.

Clear fluids as tolerated.

Ambulate twice daily.

June 4 Discontinue I.V.'s.

Bisacodyl (Dulcolax), suppository, 10 mg., now.

June 7 Fleet enema.

Soft diet.

June 8 Clamp T-tube for 4 hours; open for 2 hours during the day.

If nausea and vomiting, unclamp tube.

Leave unclamped overnight.

June 9 Remove T-tube.

Up ad lib.

Low-fat diet.

June 14 Discharge tomorrow.

NURSING INTERVENTION—POSTOPERATIVE PHASE

OBJECTIVES	APPROACH
Prevent atelectasis.	Turn, cough, and deep-breathe, q.h.; this is especially important since Mrs. Summers is obese and reluctant to move about in bed.
Prevent thrombophlebitis and atelectasis.	Ambulate morning and evening on first postoperative day.
	Apply scultetus binder prior to getting out of bed to give abdominal support.
	Pin T-tube to gown below waist; carry T-tube drainage bottle for patient.
Prevent distention.	Attach Levin tube to low suction.
	Irrigate with 20 ml. of normal saline p.r.n.
	Measure and record nasogastric drainage.
Prevent discomfort.	Give analgesic q.3-4h. as necessary to lessen pain and to ensure deep breathing and moving about in bed.
	Be sure to turn, cough, and deep-breathe Mrs. Summers about one-half hour after medication (she is most comfortable then).

NURSING INTERVENTION—POSTOPERATIVE PHASE—cont'd

OBJECTIVES	APPROACH
Prevent dislodgment of drainage tubes.	Fasten Levin tube to bed with slack between patient and edge of bed.
	Connect T-tube to I.V. tubing inserted in a 250 ml. bottle attached to bed frame.
	Turn carefully to prevent dislodging of T-tube.
Promote adequate intake and output.	Offer fluids q.1-2h.
	Record I.V. and oral intake.
	Record urinary, Levin, and T-tube drainage.
	Check daily for bowel movement.
Prevent excoriation of skin.	Check dressing frequently after T-tube is removed.
	Change dressings as necessary (heavy bile drainage is present).
	Protect skin with petrolatum gauze around T-tube.
Promote normal bowel habits.	After first bowel movement (June 5), check all stools for color, and chart.
	Discuss the importance of adequate roughage in diet.
Prepare for discharge.	Discuss need for low-fat diet.
	Have dietitian go over appropriate diets with patient.
	Encourage Mrs. Summers to rest periodically at home and to avoid heavy lifting for 6 weeks. Involve husband and children in discussions whenever possible.
	Emphasize importance of follow-up visits to her doctor.

Mrs. Summers did very well after surgery and had no episodes of nausea or vomiting even when her T-tube was clamped. At first she was reluctant to move about in bed and to ambulate, but with support and encouragement and pain medication p.r.n., she was able to move and walk more freely. After she had been out of bed for 3 days with assistance, she was able to be up and about on her own. Her sutures were removed on the sixth postoperative day, and she was transferred to the continuing care center (CCC) on the eighth postoperative day, where she remained for 4 days. The period of time in the CCC allowed her to become more independent and yet be under medical and nursing supervision. Mrs. Summers lost 10 lb. while in the hospital and was determined to lose about 20 lb. more after discharge. The nurse in charge of the CCC had the dietitian visit Mrs. Summers to discuss reduction diets with her. The nurse stressed the need to avoid "crash diets," especially while her body needed adequate protein for repair after surgery. Since Mrs. Summers' husband and teen-age children are not overweight, plans were discussed with her for modifying her own diet from the food she normally prepares for the rest of the family.

Mrs. Summers took a nap every afternoon and stated she slept well at night. Thus, when she left the hospital on her thirteenth postoperative day, she felt she could manage quite well at home, especially since her husband and children were supportive and seemed to realize her need to "take things easy" for about 6 weeks after discharge.

CHAPTER 19

HEPATIC DECOMPENSATION AND HEPATIC COMA IN A 40-YEAR-OLD WOMAN

JEAN WILLACKER

MEDICAL HISTORY AND PSYCHOSOCIAL BACKGROUND

Mrs. Clayton is a 40-year-old housewife with one teen-ager. Her husband has a good job and is interested in keeping the family healthy. The patient entered the hospital with her first grand mal seizure and occult gastrointestinal bleeding (4+ guaiac stools). This was her first admission to the hospital, and she spent 3 weeks undergoing a diagnostic work-up. During this time, she had two grand mal seizures. Since this was Mrs. Clayton's first hospitalization and her first experience with seizures, she was very frightened about what was going to happen to her. The nursing staff spent much time with her in an attempt to reduce her fear.

All diagnostic tests, including an EEG and liver biopsy, were normal and Mrs. Clayton was discharged with no special orders and was to be followed in the clinic. To provide continuity of care, the in-patient nursing staff communicated Mrs. Clayton's fears to the clinic nursing staff who would be caring for her after discharge.

One week later Mrs. Clayton returned to the clinic. At this time she had ascites, was confused mentally, and asterixis (a flapping tremor) was elicited. She was asked to calculate backwards from 100 subtracting 7 (serial 7's) and could not get any farther than 93. She was oriented to person and place but had difficulty in determining the time of day. Mrs. Clayton was aware of her mental deficiencies and was anxious because of her lack of recall.

Since Mr. Clayton wanted to take good care of his wife, he bought her expensive food, and they ate steak every day. The high-protein diet was more than her damaged liver could handle. Ammonia intoxication contributed to hepatic encephalopathy, as clinically displayed here. Ironically, her previous liver biopsy had been normal, which points to the fact that a biopsy may provide useful clinical data, but alone does not determine the diagnosis. In addition, Mrs. Clayton's history was negative for factors that usually cause liver damage.

TREATMENT
Medical therapy

20 Gm. protein diet and 1 Gm. sodium diet.

Restrict fluids to 1000 ml. daily.

Neomycin, 500 mg., q.i.d., p.o., and neomycin enema, 1 Gm., b.i.d.—nonabsorbable antibiotic that destroys bacteria that produce ammonia in the intestine.

Maalox, 30 ml., p.o., q.2h., for occult gastrointestinal bleeding.

Aquamephyton (vitamin K_1), 100 mg., I.M., daily for 3 days for low prothrombin time.

Laboratory findings

Blood ammonia, 1 mcg. (normal, up to 1).

Not all patients with hepatic encephalopathy have increased ammonia, but it is present in a significant number of cases.

Hematocrit decreased to 28 vol.% (37 to 47).

Guaiac positive stool.

Albumin decreased to 3 Gm./100 ml. (3.4 to 5).

Alkaline phosphatase increased to 20 King-Armstrong units (3 to 14)—excreted when there is blockage of bile.

Serum glutamic oxaloacetic transaminase, increased to 90 units (9 to 40; over 40 reflects cellular damage).

Prothrombin time, 40%—responsive to vitamin K.

Bilirubin, 2 mg./100 ml. (0.1 to 1).

NURSING CARE OBJECTIVES

PROBLEM	APPROACH
Low prothrombin time.	Instruct patient regarding easy bruisability.
	Tell her not to brush teeth vigorously because gums might bleed.
	Give vitamin K as ordered.
Guaiac positive stool.	Save stool, note color, and check for guaiac.
	Give antacids.
20 Gm. protein diet.	Talk with patient and family regarding diet.
	Explain relationship between a high-protein intake and hepatic coma.
	Make appointment for dietitian to see patient.
	Reinforce dietary teaching.

NURSING CARE OBJECTIVES—cont'd

PROBLEM	APPROACH
Ascites.	Measure abdominal girth daily.
	Weigh at the same time each day.
	Allow patient to help set up schedule for fluid intake.
	Provide 1 Gm. sodium diet.
Susceptibility to infection.	Maintain aseptic technique by good handwashing.
	Report any temperature elevation.
Inability of liver to detoxify certain substances.	Question orders for sedatives or central nervous system depressants that are detoxified by the liver.
Anxiety.	Explain procedures and tests to her.
	Involve family in support of patient.
Occasional disorientation.	Stay with her during periods of disorientation.
	Assess her mental status by administering specified tests.

EVALUATION OF MENTAL STATUS

The following are suggested ways to evaluate the mental orientation of a patient with a diagnosis of hepatic coma. Ideally, these questions should be asked systematically and be repeated every 8 hours. Since many patients with hepatic encephalopathy may become indignant when asked these questions, it is important that they be asked tactfully. Usually the nurse giving direct care to the patient is the best one to ask the questions. The questions may be prefaced with a remark such as: "I know these are silly questions, but by answering them you can help us in planning your care in the hospital." These questions are used to test the patient's ability to concentrate, to correlate, and to remember.

1. Orientation.
   a. Time, such as day, month, year.
   b. Place, such as hospital, home.
   c. Person, such as his name, family, nurse's name.
2. Serial 7's.
   Have patient start with 100 and work backwards subtracting 7—100, 93, 86, 79, etc.
3. Have patient write his name or a short sentence.
   A sample of his normal (premorbid) handwriting may be needed for comparison.
4. Have patient draw a five-sided star.
5. Observation of behavior and thought processes for any significant change.
6. Have patient count forwards from 1 to 10 and then backwards from 10 to 1.

7. Remote memory, such as when he was born or the names of the last three presidents.
8. Recent memory, such as name of the current president.
9. Additional observations.
   a. Asterixis (liver flap, flapping tremor). Test for asterixis by having patient flex palm of hand backward while resting his forearm on a stationary object and then instruct him to spread his fingers apart. Test is positive if patient is unable to keep hand in a fixed position.
   b. Motion of extremities.
   c. Change in muscle tone or muscle position.
   d. Restlessness.
   e. Reaction and equality of pupils.
   f. Level of consciousness.
   g. Response to stimuli.
   h. Change in vital signs.
   i. Intake and output.
10. Accurate recording of data and comparison of daily assessments to evaluate stage of coma and plan care.
11. Stages of hepatic coma.
    Stage 1—Apathy, depression, or euphoria with or without objective neurologic signs; untidy appearance; slurred speech; mild confusion; change in sleeping pattern (such as wakefulness and wandering at night).
    Stage 2—Personality changes with neurologic abnormality; inappropriate behavior.
    Stage 3—Loss of sphincter control; stuporous but responsive to stimuli; sleeps most of the time; speech incoherent.
    Stage 4—Comatose; may or may not respond to deep pain.
       As one stage progresses to another, confusion and disorientation advance.

With medical and nursing care, Mrs. Clayton began to improve. Her asterixis disappeared; urinary output increased and abdominal girth decreased. She became vibrant and acutely aware of her situation, and staff members said that she seemed more intelligent and brighter than they had ever seen her. After 2 weeks, she was discharged from the hospital.

Mrs. Clayton is being followed closely in the clinic by a doctor and a nurse clinician who cared for her in the hospital, and both will be alert for subtle change in her behavior. They have instructed the husband and daughter to watch for signs of impending coma; the husband and daughter are now well versed in regard to precipitants of coma. Mrs. Clayton has had no recurrence of coma, and her ascites has disappeared. She has a good understanding of her illness and realizes the importance of a low-protein diet to maintain liver function at an optimal level. Because of her rapid response to the prescribed regimen, there is every reason to believe that her long-term prognosis will be favorable.

CHAPTER **20**

A WOMAN IN DIABETIC KETOACIDOSIS

CAROL MITTEN

MEDICAL HISTORY

A 38-year-old black woman was admitted to the hospital with a history of nausea, vomiting, and epigastric pain of one day's duration. These symptoms followed an episode of heavy alcohol ingestion. At the time of admission, the patient was alert, restless, short of breath (respirations, 42), and was vomiting. Miss Martin had had diabetes for 6 years and usually takes 30 units (U.) of NPH insulin and 35 U. of regular insulin daily. She had omitted her insulin for the past 2 days because she was vomiting.

PSYCHOSOCIAL BACKGROUND

Miss Martin has been working as a barmaid and usually drinks heavily 1 day each week. She is single but has a preschool child who is cared for by relatives while she is at work. Miss Martin lives with her sister and the sister's family, but attempts to be financially independent in all other respects.

TREATMENT
Medical therapy

Sodium chloride, 0.45%, was begun and administered rapidly at 300 to 500 ml./hour. Crystalline insulin, 50 U., was added to the infusion. Regular insulin, 50 U., was given subcutaneously at periodic intervals thereafter. A urine specimen was obtained at the time of admission. When the patient was unable to void again after 4 hours, a Foley catheter was inserted. Urine volume, glucose, and acetone content were recorded hourly.

Vital signs were taken (temperature, 37.4° C. [99.3° F.]; pulse, 104; respiration, 42; blood pressure, 130/80) and monitored closely to determine abrupt fluctuations. A central venous pressure line was inserted and monitored closely. Since intravenous fluids were being administered rapidly (300 to 500 ml./hour), the central venous pressure readings were checked for an abrupt increase (which

122

would indicate impending congestive heart failure) or a decrease (vascular shock). Special emphasis was placed upon the depth and rate of respirations and the regularity of the pulse rate. Miss Martin's level of consciousness and degree of restlessness were also checked frequently. A nasogastric tube was inserted to reduce gastric dilatation and consequently control nausea and vomiting. Sodium bicarbonate, 2 ampules of 44.6 mEq./50 ml., was added to the intravenous fluids 3 hours after admission when the serum sodium level changed from 141 to 117 mEq./L. (normal, 136 to 145). Potassium chloride, 40 mEq., was also added to the intravenous infusion at this time because the initial serum potassium level had changed from 7.6 to 2.9 mEq./L. (normal, 3.5 to 5). Intravenous glucose, 5%, replaced the sodium chloride solution given initially when the serum glucose levels decreased substantially from 800 to 300 mg./100 ml. (normal, 80 to 120). The change in intravenous fluids was made to avoid hypoglycemia.

Laboratory findings on admission

Blood		Normal
Glucose	885 mg./100 ml.	80-120
Serum acetone	130 mg./100 ml.	0.3-2
Potassium	7.6 mEq./L.	3.5-5
Carbon dioxide	8 mEq./L.	20-28
Urine		
Glucose	5%	0
Acetone	large amount	0

Course of treatment

Two days after the initial episode of ketoacidosis had been corrected, Miss Martin was given 20 U. of NPH insulin in the morning. At noon she complained of shortness of breath, nausea, anorexia, and weakness. She was breathing deeply and her skin was warm and dry. It was assumed that she was having an insulin reaction and she was given orange juice to drink, which she subsequently vomited. Further investigation revealed glycosuria, ketonuria, and ketonemia (40 mg./100 ml.)—all signs of ketoacidosis. Thus intravenous fluids were administered and regular insulin, 20 U., was given subcutaneously. Her symptoms subsided within an hour, and no similar episodes occurred during the remainder of the hospitalization.

NURSING INTERVENTION

1. Short-term goals
   a. *Monitor patient's condition* carefully during ketoacidosis and understand

the meaning of alterations in laboratory and clinical determinations. Accurate and systematic recording of therapy and the patient's response should include:
   (1) Frequent checks of vital signs, central venous pressure readings, and state of consciousness.
   (2) Amount and type of intravenous fluids and additives.
   (3) Blood chemistry findings.
   (4) Frequent urine specimens and test for glucose, acetone, and volume.
   (5) Type and amount of medications such as insulin, potassium chloride, and sodium bicarbonate.
 b. *Be aware of possible complications.*
   (1) Hypoglycemia may occur; understand symptoms of insulin reaction, which are tachycardia, diaphoresis, tremor, and headache. If not recognized and treated, confusion, somnolence, and convulsions result.
   (2) Vascular shock may occur. An initial gradual decrease in blood pressure may be followed by an abrupt fall. Notify physician of minor decreases in blood pressure readings.
   (3) Reduction of urinary output may indicate impending shock and renal failure.
   (4) Hypokalemia may occur; recognize clinical signs of marked weakness and electrocardiogram changes—flattened or inverted T waves and a prolonged QT interval.
   (5) Gastric dilatation may be present and should be suspected if nausea, vomiting, and abdominal pain occur.
 c. *Assist in search for infectious processes.*
   (1) Examine skin, nails, and teeth for infection.
   (2) Obtain sputum specimen for culture and sensitivity.
   (3) Obtain urine specimen for culture and sensitivity.
2. Intermediate goal
   Prevent hypoglycemic or hyperglycemic reactions during early convalescence. Be alert to factors that may precipitate such reactions, such as poor dietary intake and infection. As mentioned earlier, Miss Martin experienced a ketotic episode, the symptoms of which were not accurately interpreted. The patient was given orange juice when it was assumed that she was experiencing an insulin reaction. Further investigation showed acetone present in blood and urine, and proper corrective therapy was introduced. This particular episode may have been caused by an infectious process that had not yet been diagnosed. Shortly thereafter, a dental abscess was discovered and antibiotic therapy was initiated. Correction of acetonuria and acetonemia was achieved during hospitalization.

3. Long-range goals

a. *Prevent recurrent bouts of ketoacidosis.* The course of events prior to hospitalization provided three areas in need of better understanding by Miss Martin. A review with the patient of these events was undertaken:

(1) Discussion included the dangers of heavy drinking for diabetics, which results in a high sugar intake and possibly nausea and vomiting.

(2) Decision made by the patient to eliminate insulin when vomiting; the body needs as much as, if not more insulin at this time. Reviewed following steps to take when not feeling well: continue to take usual insulin dose at prescribed times, test urine frequently, rest in bed, and drink liquids as tolerated.

(3) Discussed need to treat infections promptly since they increase the body's needs for insulin. Explained that her dental infection contributed to the ketoacidotic episode. Reminded her that all infections, even minor ones such as colds, should be treated promptly.

b. *Review important factors in self-management of diabetes.* Through informal discussions with Miss Martin about how she managed her diabetes from day to day, an evaluation of her understanding and self-care activities was possible.

(1) *Review of insulin.* Discussed the different actions of the two kinds of insulin she had been using prior to hospitalization and the need for her to eat meals at regular times. She had previously given little attention to regular meals. During the remaining convalescent days, she was encouraged to draw up and administer the prescribed insulin dose. This provided an opportunity to observe her accuracy in selecting the correct dose and her injection technique. It also offered an opportunity to discuss the sterilization procedure used at home and the importance of rotating sites of injection. Injection sites were inspected to determine whether a systematic pattern of rotation was really being followed; other possible injection sites were introduced, such as the abdomen.

(2) *Review of diet.* Miss Martin admitted to an overindulgence in sweets. She centered the conversation around her likes and dislikes and the food currently being served to her. Since she had been quite lax in prior diet management, a simplified diet with restrictions of sweets was proposed as a realistic goal for her at this time.

(3) *Review of urine testing.* It was discovered that Miss Martin understood how to test her urine for glucose content with Clinitest tablets,

but she had not done so for about 6 months: "I didn't see any need to when I was feeling okay." Reasons for testing urine were discussed: tests serve as a guide for determining a need to increase or decrease insulin dose and help gauge the state of the diabetes. Miss Martin had not tested urine for acetone previously. Since she expressed an unusually strong interest in acetone testing and stated that this "double check" made urine testing more meaningful, this procedure was incorporated into the discharge plan in an attempt to help her recognize signs of impending acidosis.

To ensure reliability of urine testing at home, routine checks were to be kept at a minimum. Three specific days of the week were chosen for urine testing and at a time convenient with her schedule. Acetone testing was to be done only when urine glucose readings were 4 + or more. Emphasis was placed on the need for Miss Martin to check her urine two or three times a day when ill to prevent future serious acidotic episodes.

Urine testing was performed and recorded by Miss Martin during the remainder of hospitalization. This provided an opportunity to evaluate her ability to interpret and record test results and to emphasize the procedure as an important facet of diabetic care.

(4) *Review of hypoglycemic and hyperglycemic reactions.* When Miss Martin experienced the second acidotic reaction several days after admission, she could not define what kind of reaction she was experiencing. It appeared that she did not recognize symptoms of hyperglycemia in herself. She was asked to describe how she felt at the time of admission and during the episode 2 days later. It was explained to her that she was experiencing a reaction to "too much sugar" in her system. Early symptoms (polyuria and polydipsia) and their relation to sugar and acetone in the urine were emphasized.

The symptoms of hypoglycemia were also reviewed. Since Miss Martin occasionally experienced severe headaches when meals were omitted, this symptom was used as an example of an impending insulin reaction. The need to carry candy in her purse was stressed, and it was explained that unconsciousness can occur rapidly from too much insulin and too little sugar and that one or two pieces of candy will quickly relieve the hypoglycemia.

(5) *Review of skin and foot care.* Miss Martin took excellent care of her skin and feet. She understood well the precautions to be followed and therefore it was not necessary to review these with her.

c. *Investigate patient's ability to maintain proper diabetic management within her life pattern.*
   (1) *Discussion about periodic drinking problem.* Why did she think it occurs? Did she seem motivated to overcome the drinking problem? If she is motivated, help her plan actions for prevention. Since Miss Martin felt her job environment contributed heavily to her drinking habit, she considered changing employment. She considered baby-sitting during the day for other people and having her own child accompany her. She did not feel that her job as a barmaid contributed to her social life and felt that better working hours would provide a more normal home life for her child and regular hours for herself. She was living with relatives and felt that they, too, would appreciate a different working arrangement.
   (2) *Preparation of meals.* What family members would plan and prepare meals? Since Miss Martin's sister was largely responsible for meals, it was suggested that the sister needed to understand Miss Martin's diet restrictions. The patient was reluctant to involve her sister in the problem. To help her feel comfortable, it was suggested that an informal discussion be held with her sister about good nutrition for the family in general. The dietitian, therefore, talked with them about good dietary habits for the whole family with emphasis on the children's needs, the patient's needs, and since they were both overweight, the benefits of weight reduction.
   (3) *Family relationship.* Because Miss Martin seemed reluctant to involve her sister in her care, it was decided that this relationship should be explored for signs of strain in the home environment. The nurse talked privately with the sister and inquired about the patient's acceptance of her condition. The sister was most receptive to an open discussion of the home situation and related that the patient tended to deny her diabetic condition in many ways. Miss Martin took her insulin, but ate sporadically and frequently ate the wrong things. The sister could not elaborate on specific areas of strain other than the patient's frustration at having to rely on relatives for help in raising her child. The sister wished to understand Miss Martin's management routine and hoped she could bring herself to talk with her more openly about it.

NURSING DISCHARGE SUMMARY
1. Plans were completed for Miss Martin to attend dental clinic for improved dental health and diabetic clinic for continued diabetic control.

2. Communication was established with nursing personnel in the out-patient clinics concerning:
   a. Aspects of diabetic care reviewed with Miss Martin.
   b. Teaching areas that may need further evaluation or emphasis.
   c. Objectives of care not fulfilled upon the patient's discharge.
   d. Books used to help Miss Martin understand her disease, which are the following:
      (1) Dolger, H., and Seeman, B.: How to live with diabetes, New York, 1965, Pyramid Publications, Inc.
      (2) Rosenthal, H., and Rosenthal, J.: Diabetic care in pictures: simplified statements with illustrations prepared for the use of the patient, ed. 4, Philadelphia, 1968, J. B. Lippincott Co.
      (3) U. S. Public Health Service, Diabetes and Arthritis Control Program: Diabetes and you, Washington, D. C. 20402, 1968, U. S. Government Printing Office (single copies free of charge).
      (4) Weller, C., and Boylan, B. R.: The new way to live with diabetes, New York, 1966, Doubleday & Co., Inc.

CHAPTER 21

NURSING NEEDS OF A SEVERELY BURNED CHILD

GLORIA A. HENDERSON

MEDICAL HISTORY

While she was attempting to warm herself at an open heater in her home, Donna's nightgown caught fire, resulting in a flame thermal injury to 41% of her body, including the anterior and posterior trunk, the buttocks, both posterior thighs, the knees and lower legs, and small areas on her arms. Twenty-three percent of her body sustained a full-thickness burn, and 18% a partial-thickness burn. Donna was admitted directly to the burn unit of a large metropolitan hospital.

PSYCHOSOCIAL BACKGROUND

Donna is a 9-year-old black female, the middle sibling of seven children between the ages of 3 and 14. They live in a low socioeconomic metropolitan area. Her parents are divorced; her mother is employed and a maternal aunt lives in the home and provides much of the child care.

INITIAL TREATMENT
Medical therapy

1. Removal of burned clothing and cleaning of the injury with sterile water and a hexachlorophene liquid soap. Concomitantly, the extent and depth of the injury was evaluated.
2. Evaluation of respiration and airway; no tracheostomy was required.
3. Venous cutdown with an 18-gauge polyethylene catheter inserted in the cephalic vein at the wrist. An intravenous infusion of lactated Ringers solution was started, calculated according to the Brooke formula. Donna's weight was estimated as 30 kg. (66 lb.).
4. Insertion of an indwelling catheter. Accurate intake and output is essential to evaluate renal function and provide an index for fluid therapy.

129

Urine specific gravity was found to be 1.022 (normal, 1.010 to 1.025), and a specimen was sent to the laboratory.

5. Vital signs, including evaluation of Donna's sensorium.
6. Culture of the wounds.
7. Morphine sulfate, 6 mg., given intravenously for sedation.
8. Tetanus toxoid, 0.5 ml., given as a booster.
9. Procaine penicillin, 600,000 U., b.i.d., given as prophylaxis against infection.
10. Application of para-[aminomethyl]benzenesulfonamide (Sulfamylon) to burn surfaces to prevent and retard bacterial invasion.
11. Exposure method of treatment of wounds. Placement of patient on sterile bed in a laminar flow unit. This unit is a special contamination-reduction system to provide for environmental isolation of patients with low resistance.

Laboratory findings

Serum electrolytes		Normal
Potassium	4.9 mEq./L.	4-5.4
Sodium	138 mEq./L.	138-148
Chlorides	99 mEq./L.	100-110
Hemoglobin	11 Gm./100 ml.	13-15.5
Hematocrit	49 vol.%	40-45
Blood urea nitrogen	15 mg./100 ml.	3-28

Nursing intervention

The initial interventions for Donna based on nursing assessment, medical therapy, and laboratory evaluation are the following:

1. Reassurance that she would survive this severe thermal injury; alleviation of her fear of the strange environment and treatments.
2. Reestablishment of fluid and electrolyte equilibrium according to physician's calculations, laboratory determinations, and observation of vital signs, intake and output, and the patient's sensorium by the nurse.
3. Judicious use of sedatives during the first 48 hours of hospitalization. Because of the anticipated prolonged hospitalization, careful assessment was made of the need for sedatives and narcotics.
4. Provision for comfort and positioning in bed to prevent contractures especially of the shoulders, hips, knees, and ankles; appropriate draping to allow exposure of wounds while maintaining patient comfort and privacy.
5. Careful evaluation of hourly intake and output (40 to 50 ml./h. is ade-

quate) and of urine specific gravity as evidence of renal function and as a basis for fluid therapy.

6. Prevention of infection through wound cleansing and application of Sulfamylon cream.
7. Specialized procedures to maintain medical asepsis, since Donna was placed in the plastic tent isolation of the laminar flow unit.
8. Reassurance of family by explaining Donna's physiologic condition and therapy in understandable terms. Encouragement of family to verbalize their feelings.

Donna was hospitalized for a period of 2 months during which her course of medical therapy was uneventful for a severely burned child. It was significant to note that she was free of burn wound sepsis, which was considered a direct result of the isolation in the laminar flow unit.

LONG-TERM TREATMENT
Medical goals

1. Maintain fluid and electrolyte balance.
2. Prevent infection by protective isolation and Sulfamylon application to wounds.
3. Encourage granulation tissue and burn-scar formation through cleaning and debridement of wounds.
4. Graft wounds with homografts and autografts as soon as feasible.

Nursing goals

The care of a 9-year-old girl in a "plastic-tent" room requires thoughtful planning of psychosocial and physiologic interventions. Some examples follow:

Psychosocial interventions
1. Establish warm, accepting attitude by nursing personnel.
2. Provide for mobilization of the patient's defenses and for appropriate channels of expression.
3. Encourage optimum independence in activities, such as feeding, turning, and assisting in her own hygiene as soon as possible.
4. Decrease sensory deprivation in the laminar flow unit through increased planned visual, auditory, tactile, and proprioceptive stimulation of appropriate play, conversation, and exercise.
5. Encourage expression of fears and acceptance of altered physical appearance; elevate child's self-esteem.
6. Provide for social and intellectual stimulation through meaningful activity and relationships.

7. Assess family attitudes and encourage realistic involvement with the child; support family in accepting Donna.

Physiologic interventions

1. Assess clinical signs and symptoms (vital signs, intake and output, sensorium, wounds) for alteration of physiologic equilibrium.
2. Prevent infection by (a) isolating the patient, (b) preventing contamination of wound by discharges from the bowel and bladder, and (c) cleaning of wounds and application of topical antibiotics.
3. Provide for patient comfort.
4. Promote optimal physical activity and prevent contractures through planned exercise and active and passive range of motion; maintain proper body positioning at all times.
5. Promote healing of grafted areas and donor sites through careful observation, positioning, cleaning, and use of dressings.
6. Provide a high protein–high carbohydrate–high vitamin diet to promote healing; provide for sufficient fluid intake to ensure fluid balance.

Donna was a challenging patient. Although medical therapy and surgical grafting were relatively uncomplicated, the care of a child in the laminar flow unit presented unusual challenges to the nurse. It required the nurse to be knowledgeable about and skillful in burn therapy. Furthermore, this resourcefulness was essential in providing a severely burned 9-year-old girl with emotional support and social stimuli that allowed her to integrate this traumatic episode into her life experience.

CHAPTER **22**

POSTOPERATIVE CARE OF A YOUNG MOTHER WITH A MASTECTOMY

ROXIE FERNELIUS

MEDICAL HISTORY

Mrs. Karen Foster, age 34, was admitted to the hospital for a breast biopsy and possible radical mastectomy. About a month ago she discovered a small lump in her right breast while bathing. Arrangements for hospitalization and surgery were made by the private physician whom she consulted. Her medical history was negative except for some premenstrual breast tenderness.

PSYCHOSOCIAL BACKGROUND

Mrs. Foster is married and the mother of a boy 10 years old and a girl 8. Her husband is the business manager of a small auto parts supply firm. They own their own home in the suburbs. Mrs. Foster is active in church and school activities and likes to garden and sew. She is a slim, dark-haired, soft-spoken young woman. Her parents who live in the city nearby are in close contact. Her mother is staying with the children during Mrs. Foster's hospitalization. Her husband and parents are supportive and concerned. They visit daily and keep in contact by phone. The many flowers and cards she has received are evidence of her family and friends' support.

TREATMENT
Laboratory findings

The results of the routine laboratory tests were within normal limits except for the hemoglobin, which was 10 Gm./100 ml. (normal, 12 to 16), and hematocrit, which was 29.5 vol.% (normal, 38 to 47).

Medical therapy

Mrs. Foster was taken to surgery after the usual preoperative preparations. A biopsy of the mass was taken and was examined immediately by means of a

133

frozen section by the pathologist, with the resulting diagnosis of cancer. The right breast, the muscles of the chest wall, and adjacent lymph nodes were then surgically removed. A drainage catheter was inserted through a stab wound into the right axilla and attached to a portable suction apparatus, the Hemovac. She was transferred to the recovery room, where her vital signs were closely monitored and her recovery was uneventful. She received 2 units of whole blood and was observed carefully for signs of reaction. There were none. Her hemoglobin increased to 13 Gm./100 ml. after transfusion and her hematocrit was 36.1 vol.%.

NURSING INTERVENTION—PREOPERATIVE PHASE

OBJECTIVES	APPROACH
To assist Mrs. Foster to cope with anxiety regarding the possible diagnosis of cancer.	Determine what the doctor has told her; allow her to express her feelings; be available for support.
To assist her in preparing for the stress of the surgical procedure.	Assess her knowledge and expectations of proposed surgery; offer explanations as needed.
To assist her with preoperative preparations.	Assess her knowledge of hospital routines; give explanations as needed.
To orient her to postoperative procedures.	Assess her knowledge of postoperative care; give explanations with each step of care.

Noting that Mrs. Foster was understandably tense and apprehensive the evening before surgery, the nurse arranged to spend time with her to offer support and assistance to help her prepare for the surgery ahead. After determining what Mrs. Foster knew about the proposed surgery and the need for preoperative preparations, the nurse explained each step as she prepared her for surgery. She also reviewed with her the postoperative nursing procedures such as turning, deep breathing, coughing, and exercises she would be asked to do after surgery. The nurse made a point of seeing Mr. Foster when he came in to visit to answer his questions and assist him as needed.

Mrs. Foster underwent surgery as previously noted. Her progress through the immediate postoperative period was uneventful. The general nursing care measures and precautions common to all patients undergoing surgery were carried out with adequate explanations at each step. Pages 135 and 136 show the specific nursing measures needed by a patient who has had a mastectomy:

NURSING INTERVENTION—POSTOPERATIVE PHASE

OBJECTIVES	APPROACH
To promote lymph drainage and venous return on affected side.	Elevate right arm, with each joint positioned higher than the more proximal joint.
	Compress Hemovac q.1h.; empty, measure, and record amount and character of drainage at end of each shift.
To promote use of arm on affected side and prevent contractures.	Passive exercises to right arm 24 hr. postoperatively per physician's order.
	Place bedside table on the right side of the bed.
	Progress to the following active exercises with right arm as physician orders:
	Hair brushing
	Hand wall climbing
	Rope turning
	Pulley motion
	Elbow pull-in
	Back scratcher
	Paddle swing
	Pendulum swing
	Forehead touch
	Relate exercises to equivalent activities of daily living.
	Encourage patient to maintain good posture.
	Use mirror to keep shoulders level
	Hold head erect
To assist her to cope with diagnosis of cancer.	Listen attentively for clues to her feelings about diagnosis.
	Allow patient to express feelings and anxieties.
	Clarify misconceptions.
To assist her to cope with anxiety about change in physical appearance.	Allow her to express her fears and concerns.
	Give valid reassurance of her feminine role.
	Provide opportunity for personal grooming
	Encourage her to maintain personal appearance by wearing own clothes as soon as possible instead of hospital gown
	Give information on prosthetic devices—temporary and permanent.
	Give explanation of the American Cancer Society's "Reach to Recovery" program, to which the physician has referred her.
	Volunteers who have had mastectomies will visit patient to give advice (nonmedical) on exercises, clothing, and prostheses
To increase sense of well-being and control of environment.	Allow her to make decisions about own care when appropriate.
	Encourage self-responsibility for doing exercises.
	Praise patient on progress made.

Continued.

NURSING INTERVENTION—POSTOPERATIVE PHASE—cont'd

OBJECTIVES	APPROACH
To assist husband and family to adjust to diagnosis of cancer and surgical procedure.	Allow husband and family to express feelings and concerns. Clarify misconceptions. Be available for support.
To assist Mrs. Foster in understanding need for follow-up care and periodic check-ups.	Find out what instructions her physician has given her. Reinforce instructions: Keep appointments with physician Elevate arm frequently Continue arm exercises, substituting household chores that are equivalent in activity Gradually resume hobbies of sewing and gardening Wear loose or nonconstricting clothing

Mrs. Foster progressed well through the postoperative recovery period. She was visibly relieved when the doctor assured her that the tumor was completely removed. Since the pathologist reported that the lymph nodes had not been invaded, no radiotherapy was contemplated. Mrs. Foster understands the importance of follow-up care and periodic check-ups.

She was discharged home on the sixth postoperative day, since she did not wish to be transferred to the continuing care center. Therefore, the doctor made arrangements for the Reach to Recovery representative to visit her at home.

CHAPTER 23

A MAN HAVING CATARACT SURGERY

ELIZABETH FORD PITORAK

MEDICAL HISTORY

Five years ago Mr. Zach had an acute myocardial infarction. His recovery was uncomplicated and, at present, he is not taking any medications. Mr. Zach wears glasses because he is nearsighted (myopic). For the past several months, he has noticed a change in his vision. Objects progressively became blurred; thus he assumed that his eyes needed to be refracted. The family physician noted that he had bilateral cataracts, but he stated that surgery was not warranted at that time. Since Mr. Zach's poor vision was increasingly interfering with activities of daily living, such as driving, he consulted an ophthalmologist. At that time, an intracapsular lens extraction (ILE) was performed on the left eye (OS). Now he has been admitted for a lens extraction of the right eye (OD).

PSYCHOSOCIAL BACKGROUND

Mr. Zach is a 48-year-old male who lives with his wife and two teen-age sons, ages 16 and 17. He is the manager of a service station. A reliable man has been employed to manage the business while Mr. Zach is in the hospital. His sons also work at the station during evenings and weekends. Mrs. Zach is not employed.

TREATMENT
Admission orders

Terpin hydrate with codeine, 8 ml., q.4h.
Dimetapp Extentab, 1, b.i.d.
Milk of magnesia, 30 ml., q.d., p.r.n.
Aspirin, 64 mg., q.4h., p.r.n. for pain.
Routine laboratory work—all results were within normal limits.

Mr. Zach has a slight upper respiratory infection accompanied by a cough. The terpin hydrate and Dimetapp Extentabs are given to control the cough, the nasal congestion, and the rhinorrhea.

Preoperative orders

Secobarbital (Seconal), 100 mg., h.s.

N.P.O. after midnight.

Codeine, 64 mg., I.M.

Hydroxyzine HCl (Atarax), 75 mg., I.M. $\left.\right\}$ 1 hour preoperatively.

NURSING INTERVENTION
Nursing care objectives prior to surgery

1. *Orient the patient to his surroundings.*
   a. After surgery, Mr. Zach will be able to distinguish only outlines of objects until he can wear his glasses, because he is aphakic in the left eye.
   b. Put the bedside stand and telephone on the left side of the bed with the telephone within easy reach.
2. *Explain to the patient the general restrictions that will apply immediately after surgery* (see physiologic explanations later).
   a. He will be permitted to roll to his unoperative side only.
   b. He must lie on his back until instructed to turn.
   c. He must remain in bed until instructed otherwise.
3. *Assess the concerns of the patient regarding surgery.* Since Mr. Zach had the same surgery 5 months earlier, he has a good understanding of the operation and of what to expect.

The operation—cataract extraction and peripheral iridectomy

The surgery was performed under local anesthesia. The seventh nerve, which supplies the orbicularis oculi muscle, was blocked. A retrobulbar block was done to block the ciliary ganglion and the nerves that innervate the rectus muscles. Intraocular surgery is not performed under a general anesthetic because nausea with vomiting may occur. Vomiting is to be avoided at all costs because intraocular pressure increases during vomiting. If intraocular pressure is increased during an operation, the contents of the eye, mainly vitreous humor, may escape through the incision. Mr. Zach stated that the surgeon had greater difficulty achieving a good nerve block this time and that he experienced more pain than before. The enzyme, alpha-chymotrypsin, was instilled into the anterior chamber of the eye to dissolve the zonules, which are too tough to separate readily in persons under 50 years of age. An intracapsular lens extraction was performed by means of cryosurgery. At the time of surgery, a peripheral iridectomy was performed. After removal of a lens, the vitreous humor can move forward, blocking the pupil and the outflow of aqueous humor. The intraocular pressure increases in the anterior chamber and glaucoma results unless a pro-phylactic iridectomy is performed.

At the termination of the surgery, the surgeon was unable to keep the eyelid closed because of the prolonged effect of the nerve block; thus it was necessary to suture it closed. The suture caused increased discomfort for Mr. Zach, but fortunately the suture was removed in 24 hours.

Postoperative orders for the day of surgery and the first postoperative day

Position on back or unoperated side.
Elevate head of bed 30 degrees p.r.n.
May stand to void.
Regular diet.
Meperidine HCl (Demerol), 50 mg., I.M., q.4h., p.r.n.
Aspirin, 64 mg., q.4h., p.r.n.
Secobarbital, 100 mg., h.s., p.r.n.
Milk of magnesia, 30 ml., p.r.n.

Nursing care objectives after surgery

1. *Prevent an increase in intraocular pressure:*
   a. Resulting from blockage of venous return in the head and neck area. Instruct Mr. Zach not to lift any heavy objects (over 1 to 2 lb.) and not to strain during bowel movements. During the act of Valsalva's maneuver, venous blood is temporarily prevented from returning to the heart; thus the venous pressure in the head and neck area is in-creased. This increases the venous pressure in the aqueous drainage channels and the scleral veins; therefore, intraocular pressure rises.
   b. Resulting from forceful squeezing of the orbicularis oculi muscle.
      (1) Instruct Mr. Zach to notify the nurse if nausea occurs. If it does occur, an antiemetic is given. If he vomits, he should not close his eyelids; the nurse will support his head and caution him not to strain.
      (2) Instruct him not to cough or sneeze and give p.r.n. medication for cough and nasal congestion as necessary. If Mr. Zach has to cough or sneeze, it is better for him to follow through with the mouth open rather than suppressing it, for suppression will cause a re-percussion in the head and eye.
      (3) Instruct Mr. Zach to always close the eyelid gently and not to squeeze the eyelid, especially when eye drops are given or when the dressing is changed.

(4) Assess whether Mr. Zach has eye pain and determine the type of pain.

    (a) Initially, when the anesthesia wears off, a burning sensation may occur.

    (b) If Mr. Zach states that it feels like "something is in his eye," the sensation is probably caused by the sutures.

    (c) Sudden severe pain may be caused by hemorrhage into the anterior chamber of the eye.

    (d) Since Mr. Zach may inadvertently squeeze the eyelids when in pain, administer the p.r.n. medication for pain before the pain becomes severe.

2. *Prevent stress on the suture line.* Instruct Mr. Zach not to bend forward because the posterior structures of the eye would then fall forward, putting pressure on the suture line.

    a. Have him wear slippers or shoes that he can slip into, rather than ones he would have to lean over to put on and tie.

    b. Instruct him to have others pick up objects from the floor for him. If he does pick up objects from the floor, he should squat or crouch down rather than stoop or bend over at the hips.

    c. Mr. Zach was placed in a Hi-Lo bed with automatic controls so that he could adjust the bed himself. If the Hi-Lo bed had not been available, he would have been cautioned not to bend over to use the bed crank.

3. *Provide for Mr. Zach's physical comfort and thus prevent complications that can be a direct result of overactivity.*

    a. Complications that can occur are the following:

        (1) Hyphema (hemorrhage into the anterior chamber).

            (a) This occurs 48 to 72 hours postoperatively.

            (b) The patient may awaken with a sudden severe pain in the eye.

            (c) It can result from the patient inadvertently squeezing the eyelid.

            (d) Put the patient in high Fowler's position so that the blood will settle to the lower part of the anterior chamber, thus preventing staining of the cornea and blockage of aqueous outflow resulting in increased intraocular pressure.

            (e) Medicate the patient for pain and notify the surgeon.

        (2) Prolapsed iris—the iris can prolapse into the wound if the patient strains.

(3) Rupture of the wound—this usually results from an injury such as that sustained in a fall, from putting pressure on the eye, or from rubbing the eye.

b. Comfort measures that also control activity are the following:

(1) Complete care during the time Mr. Zach is on bed rest. This includes a bath, mouth care, very gentle brushing of the teeth, and gentle hair combing. Also, feed him until he can be in high Fowler's position. Then the overbed table can be raised high so that he will not need to bend his head forward while eating.

(2) Shave him on the third postoperative day as ordered by the surgeon. Patients should not be shaved without the written order of the surgeon because jerky movements of the face during shaving can cause damage to the eye.

(3) Instruct him to avoid all jerky movements of the head.

(4) Encourage him to carry out range of motion of all extremities every 2 or 3 hours while on bed rest. Teach him to do dorsiflexion and plantar flexion of the feet; this improves venous return to the heart and prevents stasis of blood, which sometimes causes thrombophlebitis.

(5) Give him back care during the bath, at midafternoon and at bedtime. This is comforting to him since he had some arthritic changes of the spine.

(6) Offer him a glass of water or other fluid every 2 hours, in addition to fluids that he takes with meals. Lifting the water pitcher requires straining; therefore remove it from the bedside while he is on bed rest (during the first 2 postoperative days).

Orders for the second postoperative day

Out of bed with help.
House diet.
Petrogalar, 30 ml., h.s., p.r.n.

Short-term nursing care objectives in addition to earlier objectives

1. Assist Mr. Zach with activities of daily living to prevent overactivity.

   a. Always wash his legs even though he is permitted out of bed so that he will not have to bend his head forward.

   b. Plan schedule whereby Mr. Zach is up in the chair for 30 to 60 minutes. His activity will be increased as tolerated.

2. Provide for Mr. Zach's safety.

    a. Keep all doors either completely open or closed, since he can only see the outline of objects and lacks peripheral vision.

    b. Teach him to grasp the arm of the person walking with him so that the person walks slightly ahead of him, guiding his way.

    c. Help him plan his menu and include juices such as prune juice to aid in elimination.

    d. Give him Petrogalar daily unless he has a bowel movement.

Long-term nursing care objectives

1. *Assess the amount of knowledge Mr. Zach has from his previous surgery.*
     a. After his lens extraction 5 months ago, he was not permitted to do any heavy lifting for 2 months. Prior to that time he had been active in an exercise program that he had to forego for 2 months.
     b. He wore sunglasses the first few days because of photophobia. The surgeon instructed him to take aspirin for eye discomfort, but he did not find this necessary.
     c. He was fitted with temporary cataract glasses approximately 3 weeks postoperatively. Some of the adjustments to the glasses were:
       (1) Everything was magnified (approximately 30%).
       (2) Peripheral vision was lost. To see clearly, he had to look through the center of the lens. It was necessary to turn his head to see objects in the usual peripheral fields.
       (3) Movements, particularly fine ones that required depth perception and coordination, were difficult. Initially, he found it hard to judge distance when parking or backing up a car.
       (4) A blind spot was present in his peripheral visual field. On two different occasions, he almost walked in front of a moving car when he was working at the service station. As a result, he learned to compensate for this blind spot by turning his head to check what was present in his peripheral visual field.
       (5) The surgeon told him that straight lines such as door casings might appear curved, but he did not experience this.

2. *Consult with the surgeon regarding the discharge instructions.*
     a. His restrictions are the same as those after the first lens extraction. Since a detached retina is a possible complication of a lens extraction, it is extremely important that Mr. Zach not lift anything for 2 months and that he not be overactive. Retinal detachment also occurs more frequently in persons who are myopic than in those who are not, and Mr. Zach is myopic.

b. Reinforce the earlier teaching.

c. Mr. Zach was cautioned about the loss of depth perception that can occur when he is using only one eye. He was accustomed to looking down at the first step before descending stairs. Now he must be extra cautious, as he should not bend his head downward during the healing process.

d. He is to wear an eye patch for the first week. Mr. Zach and his wife were taught to apply the eye patch as follows: Close the eye gently. Secure the patch with two pieces of Scotch tape applied diagonally from the forehead to the cheek.

e. At all other times he should wear his regular glasses. Mr. Zach hopes to be fitted with contact lenses since they provide a better refraction and objects are magnified only 5%, rather than 30% as occurs with cataract lenses.

f. Mr. Zach and his wife were taught to wash their hands before touching the eye. When the eye needs to be cleaned, cotton balls moistened with water that has been boiled for 10 minutes and cooled should be used. They were taught how to wipe from the inner corner of the eye to its outer corner without putting pressure on the eye.

3. *Determine whether Mr. Zach and his wife understand the instructions and whether they have any questions that need to be answered.*

a. Both Mr. and Mrs. Zach seemed to understand the restrictions and why they were necessary. He was reminded not to drive a car.

b. On the day of discharge, Mrs. Zach came to pick up her husband. She was very protective of him. While she was packing his suitcase, she had him sit in a chair and made certain that he did not bend over to tie his shoes. She did not permit him to lift the suitcase.

c. Mr. Zach was given an appointment to see the doctor in 2 weeks and was instructed to consult his physician prior to that time if he experienced unusual discomfort.

CHAPTER 24

A YOUNG WOMAN WITH AN ACUTE, SEVERE, EXACERBATION OF MULTIPLE SCLEROSIS

MARGARET A. PALERMO

MEDICAL HISTORY

Three months prior to the present admission, Miss Daniels was hospitalized after the abrupt onset of blurred vision, with a decrease in visual acuity and pain in her right eye. The condition was diagnosed as an optic neuritis of the right eye (OD). After a 2-week course of ACTH gel (40 U., b.i.d., I.M.), her vision improved considerably, and although still not normal, she was discharged and returned to work.

Three weeks after this discharge, Miss Daniels was readmitted with the same complaint; this time, however, both eyes were affected. She stated that the fluorescent lights at work bothered her eyes so that she had to wear sunglasses and that at times her legs "felt like rubber." Physical examination revealed that she was unable to distinguish colors; the left pupil was 1 mm. larger than the right, and both pupils were reactive to light and accommodation. She was unable to see the central dot laterally on the Amsler grid. She demonstrated increased muscle tone and decreased strength in her left upper extremity and three-beat clonus of her left ankle. The symptoms indicated a bilateral retrobulbar neuritis, but this was interpreted as a manifestation of the syndrome of multiple sclerosis. After 10 days, Miss Daniels began to demonstrate some return of visual acuity, but the recovery was not complete. During this time, she also developed numbness and paresthesia in her trunk and occasionally in her legs and hands. She had occasional difficulty in walking, concomitant with the sensory changes in her legs. Four weeks after admission, she was discharged ambulatory. However, she still had difficulty in seeing and recognizing images, and the numbness and occasional paresthesias of her trunk and thighs persisted.

During the week after the patient's discharge, her vision continued to improve, but she began having extensor spasms of her legs, fell several times as a result of this, could barely walk, and was readmitted on the seventh day. The fingers on both hands were numb, and she demonstrated some clumsiness when attempting to use her right hand. She had no disturbances in sphincter control (urinary or bowel), but did have decreased ability to postpone voiding. On physical examination, she was described as a "Cushingoid young woman, markedly tearful and depressed."

Miss Daniels' neurologic symptoms continued to progress rapidly, and she developed spasms of the abdominal muscles, more painful extensor and flexor spasms of the right leg (and eventually the left leg), decreased hand grasp, increased spasticity of the upper extremities (with eventual flexor spasms of the right arm and hand), and by the tenth day a complete quadriplegia. Urinary retention developed, and voluntary control of the anal sphincter was lost. At this point, her condition stabilized. It was several weeks before muscular spasms became less frequent and some voluntary motor activity began to return. Three months after the beginning of the third hospitalization, the patient walked out of the hospital, unassisted, and 2 months later was back at work full-time with no apparent neurologic deficits.

PSYCHOSOCIAL BACKGROUND

Carol Daniels is a 24-year-old "career girl" who is employed as a fabric buyer for a large fashion house. She shares an apartment with one of her co-workers. She is a college graduate and also attended a fashion school for 1 year after her college graduation. She has one sister who lives in the same city; her parents have retired and are living in Florida. She is an avid skier, both on snow and water, and spends much of her free time in pursuit of these activities.

For ease in presentation, the medical therapy, laboratory data, and nursing intervention are discussed together. Since the course of this patient's illness is prolonged, the discussion is divided into three stages. The initial acute stage occurred when voluntary muscular function was decreasing. During the "plateau" phase muscular function was at a minimum and the prognosis very uncertain. The rehabilitative phase covered the time when voluntary muscular function began to return until she was discharged from the hospital.

ACUTE PHASE
Medical therapy

On admission
ACTH gel, 40 U., I.M., q.3d.
Azathioprine (Imuran), 50 mg., p.o., q.i.d.
KCl, 0.32 mg., p.o., b.i.d.

Maalox, 30 ml., t.i.d.
Histamine, 2.75 mg. in 250 ml. of normal saline, I.V., q.d. for 8 days
Diazepam (Valium), 5 mg., p.o., t.i.d.
Codeine, 32 mg., with aspirin 640 mg., q.4h., p.r.n. for pain
Up ad lib; assist as necessary
Later
Hypothermia blanket continuously
Discontinue codeine
Pentazocine lactate (Talwin), 50 mg., I.M. q.4h., p.r.n.

Laboratory findings

Cerebral spinal fluid (CSF) protein, 50 mg./100 ml. (normal, 15 to 45)
    Cells, 35/mm.^{3}, all mononuclear
        Gamma globulin, 5.2 mg./100 ml. (normal, 3 to 13)
Urinalysis, within normal limits
Urine culture and sensitivity, no growth
ECG, essentially normal

Nursing intervention

Initially, what seemed to be the most important aspects of Miss Daniels' care were related to her physical safety and her emotional reactions to the illness. The two are interrelated. This was her third hospitalization in 2 months: her vision was still much decreased; she had fallen several times at home and seemed to be losing control of her legs, which "jumped a lot"; and she cried easily. "I just can't control myself," she said and would ask, "What is happening to my body? Why is it doing this?" She knew that her original problem was "optic neuritis," but had not been told that she had multiple sclerosis. Since she had met other young persons in the hospital with multiple sclerosis who had been emotionally defeated by the knowledge of the diagnosis, the physician believed that it would be better for her not to know what she had. (Her family, however, had been told and had done a great deal of reading about the disease.) She needed answers to her questions and someone to talk to about what she was going through. The situation was discussed with the resident physician and then with her private physician, and it was decided that the resident should discuss her illness with her without giving it a name. This action seemed to reduce some of the apprehension that "nobody knew what was wrong" and gave the nursing staff the basic framework within which they could help Miss Daniels cope with her illness.

Miss Daniels was a very independent person; she would "rather do it herself" and did not like to ask for help. With her poor vision, the unpredictable muscular spasms in her legs, and the increasing muscular weakness and ataxia, she needed to be prevented from injuring herself by falling or bumping into objects and (a few days after admission) from spilling hot ashes or hot liquids. Her lack of sensation below the midchest level potentiated the danger, especially since she enjoyed smoking after meals. Necessary safety precautions, such as not getting out of bed by herself and smoking only when someone was with her, were discussed with Miss Daniels. To help her adjust to imposed limitations, the nursing staff made attempts to answer her light promptly, offered to stay with her so that she could smoke, and offered to help her get up. She was encouraged to do things for herself as long as she was able, but as bathing and then feeding herself became increasingly difficult, these were done for her. The transition was not an easy one. She refused help initially, struggling along by herself and doing less each day. Only after several days did she accept the nurse's offer to help.

With the decrease in muscle strength, the frequency and intensity of the muscular spasms in the patient's lower extremities increased. The spasms in the right leg were severe. They were primarily flexor spasms of the hip and knee joints, lasting 30 seconds to 1 minute. There did not appear to be any particular situation or position that precipitated them, and they occurred quite irregularly. It was necessary to provide measures to minimize or alleviate the spasms and the pain that they produced. Diazepam, 5 mg., three times a day was ordered, as well as codeine, 32 mg., with aspirin, 640 mg., every 4 hours p.r.n. As the spasms became more painful, pentazocine was substituted for the codeine and aspirin, with greater effectiveness. Range of motion exercises and massaging the leg muscles also appeared to be effective in alleviating the spasms once they began, as did holding the legs in either a completely flexed or fully extended position. It was thought that muscular motion or massage would help reduce the muscular contraction of the spasm.

Small doses of intravenous histamine were also tried to prevent the progression of the disease, and the development of spasms. To prevent the occurrence of side effects (such as hypotension and severe headache), the histamine was administered over a 2-hour period, with frequent (q.15min. × 4, and then q.30min.) monitoring of vital signs and blood pressure. The most uncomfortable side effects were a flushed face, a rash, and an increase in the nasal and lacrimal secretions. The rate of infusion was decreased slightly if the side effects became too unbearable for the patient.

Hypothermia was also used to help prevent muscular spasms. Body temperature was lowered to 35.5° C. (95.9° F.). Since only one hypothermia blanket was used, a sheet covered Miss Daniels to prevent her from shivering. She needed to be turned every 30 minutes to prevent any body area from becoming "frozen" and completely interfering with peripheral circulation. This treatment was not as effective as anticipated and was discontinued after several days.

The control and treatment of the muscular spasms remained a problem during most of the acute stage of Miss Daniels' illness. The combination of massage and range of motion, an analgesic, and a mild muscle relaxant seemed the most effective.

Observations related to circulation, respiration, and elimination were also necessary during this period to maintain their "normal" status. As Miss Daniels became less and less able to turn and move herself, she needed to be turned frequently to prevent the development of areas of cutaneous ischemia (she also was not eating much and was slightly overweight when she was admitted) and a hypostatic pneumonia. Her legs were wrapped with elastic bandages from toes to thigh to promote the return of venous blood to the heart. She was encouraged to take deep breaths when she was turned. For convenience, range of motion exercises were done to the upper extremities and ankles at this time. With the rapid advance of paralysis, it was feared that the respiratory muscles might be affected. So, for a period of several days, respiratory rate was counted every hour, and a respirator (iron lung) was on the floor in the event of a respiratory arrest.

Miss Daniels was having some difficulty moving her bowels and in delaying urination when she felt the urge to void. The latter problem was handled by responding promptly to her requests for the bedpan. The bowel problem was slightly more complicated. She was started on a routine of prune juice and a laxative, but this was not immediately effective. A soapsuds enema was given, with excellent results, and she was then started on a daily regimen of bisacodyl (Dulcolax) tablets. She soon lost voluntary control of the rectal sphincter and had no sensation to signal her when she needed to defecate. She felt she was not able to use the bedpan and frequently requested to be helped up to the commode. This was done until she was no longer able to sit by herself and became dizzy when in an upright position.

Eight days after admission, she developed urinary retention. Bethanechol chloride (Urecholine chloride), 20 mg., p.o., was given to relax the urinary sphincter but was not effective, and she was catheterized; 850 ml. of urine was removed. Since she still was unable to void the next day, a retention catheter was inserted and attached to a closed drainage system. Observations regarding color, clarity, and amount of urine were made, and daily specimens for culture and sensitivity were obtained.

These changes occurred quite rapidly, and as painful muscular spasms increased and voluntary control of body movements decreased, Miss Daniels became more demanding and insistent that if we did not help her she would do it by herself. She was "uncomfortable" in any position except flat on her back. She insisted a light be kept on at night; she was frightened and unable to comprehend what was happening to her. With the rapidity and severity of the onset, no one *could* be sure of the prognosis. But at best, it was guarded.

The nursing approach to the patient depended on her mood. Attempts were made to respond immediately when she called. If the nurse was busy with another patient, she told Miss Daniels that she would be there in a minute. Miss Daniels didn't accept this answer and became very impatient. Extra time was spent with her—giving her something to drink, letting her smoke a cigarette, repositioning her arms and legs, rubbing her back. Sometimes she dozed off, but her sleep was often disturbed by muscle spasms. She talked about herself, the things she liked to do, and everything she was missing by being sick. She would ask what she had done to deserve this illness, but usually would end with "I'll walk out of here! You'll see!"

PLATEAU PHASE
Medical therapy

Foley catheter with closed-system drainage.

Irrigate Foley with 60 ml. normal saline p.r.n.

Urinalysis q.d.

Urine for culture and sensitivity q.d.

Daily complete blood count.

Wrap legs to thighs.

Elevate head of bed 30 degrees; if angle is tolerated, take her to T.V. room on cart.

Physical and occupational therapy—consult and treat.

Ampicillin, 500 mg., q.6h., p.o.

Trimeprazine tartrate (Temaril), 2.5 mg., p.o., q.6h., p.r.n. for itching.

Prochlorperazine dimaleate (Compazine), 5 mg., p.o., q.12h. for nausea and vomiting.

Methenamine mandelate (Mandelamine), 1 Gm., q.i.d., p.o.; discontinue ampicillin.

Diazepam, 5 mg., q.6h., p.r.n., I.M., for spasms.

Nystatin (Mycostatin) suppository (vaginal) 600,000 U., b.i.d., for 1 week.

Diazepam, 5 mg., p.o., q.i.d.; discontinue I.M. diazepam.

Nitrofurantoin (Furadantin), 50 mg., p.o., t.i.d.; discontinue Mandelamine.

Ascorbic acid, 500 mg., p.o., t.i.d.

Oxycodone HCl (Percodan), 1, q.4h., p.r.n. for pain and flexor spasms.

Laboratory findings

Urine for culture
    and sensitivity, >100,000 enterococci   } sensitivity to ampicillin and
                    >100,000 *Enterobacter aerogenes*   nitrofurantoin.

Urine for culture
    and sensitivity, >100,000 swarming proteuses.
                    sensitive to acetyl sulfasoxazole and resistant to ampicillin.

Vaginal scrapings, >100,000 *Escherichia coli* and *Enterobacter aerogenes*.
    Candida present.

Chest X-ray film, clear.

ECG, within normal limits.

Nursing intervention

During this phase of her illness when the progressive loss of voluntary muscle action stabilized, Miss Daniels was unable to move any of her extremities. She had developed a urinary tract infection for which she was given ampicillin. After 3 days of treatment, it was noted during her bath that the labia minora were quite swollen and that there was a moderate amount of white, cheesy drainage. A specimen of the drainage was obtained and sent for culture and sensitivity testing. It was thought that this was a *Candida* (*Monilia*) infection secondary to antibiotic therapy, and since the urinary tract infection was not responding to treatment by ampicillin, methenamine mandelate was substituted. Laboratory reports several days later confirmed the presence of *Candida,* and Nystatin vaginal suppositories were ordered.

Therapeutic doses of ampicillin frequently result in excessive reproduction of *Candida.* It is possible for either mucocutaneous or systemic candidiasis to develop in certain persons receiving this medication, especially those who are malnourished or debilitated, or those who are receiving steroids.[1] Since Miss Daniels had not been eating well and had been receiving ACTH, it was not strange that she did develop candidiasis. Because of the loss of sensation below her arms, she was unaware of the usual perineal itching and burning on urination that frequently accompanies vaginal infections. It is only with careful observations by the nurse that such side effects of medications can be identified.

The major nursing care problem during this time was the patient's behavior. Miss Daniels had been immobilized for nearly 3 weeks. Her visual acuity was still quite decreased (she could not recognize people when they were 1 to 2 meters away), and she continued to have painful spasms of her legs and arms. She also began to have peculiar sensations in her arms and legs, described by her as feeling as though they were "all bent up," were hanging over the edge of the bed, and were heavy, when in actuality they were straight out in front of her. She was very demanding: she commanded people to do things for her, got extremely agitated when they did not comply immediately, and began refusing to eat. When it was suggested to her that she be lifted out of bed onto the cart for a change of environment, she refused that, too. At least one study indicates that impairment in behavior under these conditions is not unusual.[2] Voices—her own and others—were her only perceived contact with others. She could not feel, move, or see. Her life depended on others taking care of those functions she often performed automatically, half consciously. Her only way of being sure that others knew of her helplessness was by telling them, and her continual calling for a drink of tea or a cigarette was her way of assuring that attention.

Members of the nursing staff began to resent Miss Daniels' constant demands. They began to walk by her room without saying anything for fear they would have to go in and would ignore her calling. When they answered her call, irritation could be heard in their voices, and the atmosphere became tense. Something had to be done. Informal conferences were held with small groups of nursing staff. The reasons for the patient's behavior were discussed, along with some projection of what she might be feeling, and the staff's hostile feelings were aired. Plans were made for daily discussions as necessary. Gradually, the tension diminished. A plan of care was instituted to try to set some limits for Miss Daniels and to increase her trust in the staff's ability to meet her needs. The first step was to set up the call-light cord across the bed at face level so that she could reach it with her teeth. This was something besides calling verbally that *she* could do, and it worked well. Concomitantly, her vision began to show remarkable improvement, and she began to have some return of sensation in her arms and, within a few days, some movement. These changes had a noticeable effect on the patient's behavior. She became less insistent and would agree to wait for her drink of water or cigarette. The staff checked frequently to see whether she wanted anything and told her when they were leaving and when they would return. They found this, along with a calm unhurried approach, to be effective. She began to ask to have her records or the radio on and began to joke with the staff and visitors.

Miss Daniels' physical nursing care during this time was directed toward maintaining normal functional ability. Measures were taken to prevent foot drop, contractures of hands and wrists, decubiti, and other hazards of immobility. Since she was unable to sit upright without becoming dizzy, a program of gradual, day by day elevation of the head of the bed was instituted in preparation for getting her into a wheelchair. As soon as she could tolerate being up 45 degrees, steps were taken to get her into a reclining wheelchair. It took Miss Daniels several days to adjust to the idea of getting up. She was only able to stay up 15 minutes the first time, but within a few days she was able to stay up for 1 hour. The occupational therapist was asked to evaluate her ability to feed herself. Miss Daniels now had gross muscular movements in her right hand and arm. With the use of a movable armrest, a long straw, a plate guard, and silverware with built-up handles, she was able to feed herself. However, she needed a great deal of encouragement to try during the first few weeks, and she frequently refused (because she "made such a mess") to do anything but move her head into position for using the straw. As she regained more and more use of her arms and hands, she became much more eager to try new things. These successful attempts and her intense determination not to become an invalid created the motivation needed for rehabilitation.

REHABILITATION PHASE
Medical therapy

Bisacodyl suppositories, 1, and Dulcolax tablets, 1, a.c. (breakfast), every other day.

Nystatin vaginal tablets, 100,000 U., 1, q.d.

Aspirin, 640 mg., q.4h., p.r.n., for pain.

Darvon capsules, 65 mg., 1 q.4h., p.r.n., for pain if aspirin not effective.

Nysta-Dome lotion to perineum, t.i.d. for 10 days.

Keep legs apart; infrared lamp for 15 min. q.i.d.

Begin clamping Foley catheter for 1 or 2 h. as tolerated and drain for 10 min.

Laboratory findings

Urine culture and sensitivity, no growth.

Nursing intervention

The primary objective of nursing care during this phase of Miss Daniels' illness was to encourage *as much independence as she could possibly attain.* The major areas of concern were activities of daily living, elimination, and her psychosocial adjustment to her limitations. However, the *Candida* infection still remained a problem. To control the infection, nystatin vaginal tablets and Nysta-Dome lotion were used. Heat was applied to the perineum to decrease the soreness and inflammation of the labia, and her legs were kept apart to decrease mechanical irritation of the edematous labia.

The goal with relation to elimination was to regain normal bowel and bladder function, within physiologic limits. A regimen of bisacodyl suppositories and bisacodyl tablets was begun in the morning every other day, and a Foley catheter clamping routine was instituted. The former was successful in preventing constipation and in establishing a regular pattern. Gradually, the medication was reduced to one tablet at bedtime with prune juice and plenty of fruits and vegetables in her diet. It is important not to create a dependency on laxatives as long as natural regulation can be obtained. The Foley clamping routine was instituted to overcome the atony of the bladder—a condition that usually occurs with prolonged use of a catheter. It may take several weeks for the bladder walls to regain their tone. Initially, the catheter is clamped for 1 or 2 hours and then drained for 10 to 15 minutes. The patient's tolerance of the clamping is evaluated in terms of whether the patient can feel pressure and thus has the desire to void and whether there is evidence of urine leaking around the catheter. If neither of them occurs while the catheter is clamped, the time is gradually increased (every two or three days) until the patient can tolerate clamping for about 4 hours. Miss Daniels had difficulty when the catheter was first clamped and could only tolerate clamping for one-half hour. After 2 weeks, the catheter could be clamped for 4 hours without discomfort and it was removed. Observations made after the catheter was removed included (1) how long she remained continent and (2) whether she could void by herself when she had the desire. She had no difficulty with either incontinence or retention once the catheter was removed.

Progress in activities of daily living paralleled increasing muscular function. Miss Daniels was encouraged to do as much as she could for herself in bathing and eating. The physical therapist worked closely with her to improve her ability to sit, stand, and walk. The occupational therapist worked with her in redeveloping hand strength and coordination. She practiced writing and made a variety of small articles requiring gross and fine hand movements, and hand-eye coordination. Her vision was nearly normal. She accepted help when it was offered, but occasionally would try physical activities on her own that could have been more safely done with supervision.

Emotionally, she was quite optimistic. She began making plans to go home and, eventually, to return to work. She refused to baby herself and was not going to be "ruled" by her disease (she had finally found out her diagnosis); she refused to live in fear of having an exacerbation. If it came, she would face it then, but for now she was well. Her optimism was fairly realistic, for she had been told that since she had made such a complete recovery, it could be years before she would have another attack. As she made her plans to go home (first to stay with a family friend until she could leave the city and join her parents), she was confident that within 3 months she would be able to manage on her own. She did!

REFERENCES
1. Meyler, L., and Herxheimer, A.: Side effects of drugs, Baltimore, 1968, The Williams & Wilkins Co., vol. 6.
2. Zubek, J. P., Bayer, L., Milstein, S.., et al.: Behavioral and physiological changes during prolonged immobilization plus perceptual deprivation, J. Abnorm. Psychol. 74:230-236, April 1969.

CHAPTER 25

A MAN WITH PARKINSON'S DISEASE

CAROLYN BINGHAM DAVIS

MEDICAL HISTORY

Mr. Baker, age 67, has had Parkinson's disease for the past 12 years. His symptoms have progressed until he is now moderately disabled and requires assistance in personal care. His physician recommended that a nurse from the Visiting Nurse Association (VNA) evaluate the home situation to assess the effect and tolerance of Mr. Baker to levodopa (a new medication for Parkinson's disease) and to help the patient and his wife learn ways of coping with his disability.

The VNA nurse first visited the week before Mr. Baker was started on levodopa. She found that Mr. Baker had akinesia, described by him as "trouble getting myself going." He felt this caused the most problems in performing daily functions, since he had impaired ability to initiate, terminate, and vary his movements. The nurse observed the effects of the akinesia by asking him to transfer from bed to chair, to walk across the room, and then to turn into the kitchen. After a delay in getting started, he found it hard to turn at the precise time for the doorway and to stop without going too far. He walked by leaning forward and shuffling in small steps and reported that he often "froze" while walking and had considerable difficulty getting started again. He told her that at night he had trouble turning in bed.

Rigidity was detected when the nurse performed range of motion exercises. Other typical features of Parkinson's disease were present: a fixed staring expression, a closed jaw, and compressed lips. His speech was usually monotonous in quality, but at times it became quite rapid and tended to become more rapid as he continued to talk. As his speech increased in rate, the volume decreased. A "rest tremor" was seen in his fingers when he was in a relaxed position. It disappeared when he performed voluntary movements such as feeding himself, but as he continued eating, the tremor sometimes reappeared and caused him to spill fluids or food. Mr. and Mrs. Baker said that they rarely ate out now because of his embarrassment about being messy in front of others.

The combination of these symptoms made it difficult for Mr. Baker to accomplish fine motor tasks that the nurse had him demonstrate: buttoning clothing, tying shoelaces, and putting on a necktie. He reported that his wife frequently had to do these things for him, particularly if he did not have unlimited time to get dressed. When the nurse asked him for a handwriting sample, he was slow to start the first letter, and as he went on, the letter size gradually diminished and then trailed off into a wavy line.

MEDICAL THERAPY

Mr. Baker was taking trihexyphenidyl HCl (Artane), 2 mg., t.i.d., which he felt had some beneficial effect on his rigidity, but none on his disinclination to move. The drug's atropine-like effect had also alleviated his tendency to drool. A higher dosage of 4 mg., t.i.d., prescribed earlier was reduced to the current schedule since he experienced excessive dryness of the mouth, urinary retention, confusion, and hallucinations. He had been frequently constipated since the symptoms of Parkinson's disease began, and high dosages of trihexyphenidyl HCl tended to make this worse.

Mr. Baker was started on 250 mg. of levodopa, b.i.d. The dosage was to be increased by 250 mg. and later by 500 mg. every third day as tolerated, until maximum effect was achieved with no adverse side effects. During the regulation of the dosage of levodopa, Mr. Baker visited his physician at the office once a week and was seen by the VNA nurse every other day for 2 weeks, twice a week until the dose was stabilized, and then p.r.n. She telephoned reports to the physician to discuss any changes in the patient's symptoms and also any excessive side effects. In this way the doctor could adjust the dosage as necessary until a therapeutic level, usually between 3 and 7 Gm. a day, was reached.

NURSING INTERVENTION

Since anorexia, nausea, and vomiting are frequent and expected side effects of levodopa, the nurse instructed the patient to take the medication at the end of a meal or a snack, such as after a glass of milk, toast, crackers, or some other bland food. One-half ounce of an antacid, such as magnesium aluminum hydrate (Riopan), was sometimes taken with between-meal doses. Since Mr. Baker knew he should not take the medicine on an empty stomach, he took his 4 Gm. a day as follows: 1 Gm. at the end of lunch and supper and 500 mg. after breakfast and after a snack at midmorning, midafternoon, and early evening. He kept a calendar taped to the refrigerator door with his daily dosage schedule (which was particularly valuable during the weeks the dosage was gradually being increased), and his wife poured out the total dose for the day in an egg cup that they kept at his place at the table. When he first started the between-meal doses, he set an alarm clock for the prescribed times so that he could remember to take his snack and medication.

His first side effect, nausea, occurred while he was taking 2 Gm. of levodopa. The physician and nurse had discussed the expected gastrointestinal effects with him, and so he continued to take the prescribed doses that day after small amounts of food. He vomited suddenly after breakfast the next morning. The first dose for that day was lost, but he was able to eat a light lunch and take the next dose. The nurse visited that afternoon and reported this to the physician. He ordered the dosage held at 2 Gm. for the next 4 days (if tolerated) and then increased the dosage to 2.5 Gm. in five divided doses. These periods of nausea and vomiting continued intermittently for the next 3 weeks, but Mr. Baker was determined to continue the drug if possible. The nurse suggested to Mrs. Baker that she prepare small, more frequent amounts of food of his choice, omitting highly seasoned and fried foods. The nurse kept the doctor informed about the patient's episodes of significant emesis so the dosage could be increased or decreased as tolerated. After 6 weeks, he was able to tolerate 5 Gm. a day (1.25 Gm. after meals, 500 mg. with midmorning and midafternoon snacks, and 250 mg. with an evening snack) with very infrequent gastrointestinal problems.

The nurse took Mr. Baker's blood pressure in lying and standing positions on each visit and questioned him concerning any dizziness upon standing, since orthostatic hypotension is one of the side effects of levodopa. He reported occasional light-headedness upon arising in the morning; so she cautioned him to sit up very slowly, to sit on the side of the bed for several minutes, and then to stand in place by the bed before walking around. His systolic blood pressure dropped from an average of 170 to 145 after his dosage of levodopa reached 4 Gm. per day, but his diastolic remained between 80 and 90 and he had no further symptoms. After 6 weeks of therapy, there was no significant difference in blood pressure taken in either position.

The other side effect from levodopa was the appearance of involuntary movements that did not begin until 2 months after therapy was started. Mrs. Baker noted that her husband had wobbly movements of his head, particularly when he was doing something, such as eating or dressing. The movements often became worse when he talked or used his hands. The physician observed this on his next visit, but since it was not bothersome to Mr. Baker, the drug dosage was kept at 5 Gm. per day. He could receive a reduced dose if the movements became worse, but some of the therapeutic effect of the drug might be lost.

The patient's apical pulse was taken at each visit by the nurse, and serial electrocardiograms were taken when he saw the physician to detect any arrhythmias or changes. His blood count, blood urea nitrogen, enzymes, and urinalysis remained within normal limits. The nurse also watched for any personality or behavioral changes (such as paranoid ideation, agitation, hallucinations, and delusions), which are sometimes seen early in the course of treatment with levodopa. Mr. Baker experienced none of these behavioral side effects.

Mrs. Baker was the first one to notice the improvement in her husband's speech and facial expression. He was taking 4 Gm. of levodopa at the time. He was still having some periods of nausea and vomiting on this dosage, and since these gastrointestinal symptoms often lessen with continued use of levodopa, the nurse encouraged him to continue trying to retain the medicine and eat what he could.

The nurse also encouraged Mr. Baker to walk as much as possible and to practice rising from a chair several times a day. She taught him to do active range of motion exercises, emphasizing shoulder and hip movements and finger and wrist extension. He was taught to practice swinging his arms from flexion to hyperextension as he walked to regain some of his natural rhythm in walking. She taught him to practice handwriting by making two or three letters at a time in normal or larger than normal size, then pausing, and starting again— rather than letting the writing "freeze." Since he was more prone to falls (and fractures) as his mobility improved and he no longer sat at home or stayed in bed most of the day, the nurse cautioned both the patient and his wife about taking safety measures.

In 4 months Mr. Baker was felt to have achieved significant benefit from levodopa; he could tolerate 5 Gm. per day with no major side effects. The gastrointestinal symptoms decreased to only occasional anorexia or nausea. He had definite improvement in initiating, varying, and terminating his movements and walked almost normally. He had retired because of disability 5 years before, but now he could work in his yard and walk to nearby stores. He could dress himself without assistance and could get in and out of the tub. A slight degree of rigidity and most of the tremor remained, but he was neater while eating. He could cut his own food and open cartons. His face was less "masked," his voice was slightly more expressive, and his handwriting was more legible. He now saw his physician once a month, and VNA services were discontinued after the first 3 months.

CHAPTER 26

EVALUATION OF A MAN HAVING SEIZURES

CAROLYN BINGHAM DAVIS

MEDICAL HISTORY

Mr. Lawrence, age 35, was brought to the emergency room by ambulance after his wife found him in a stuporous state, following three grand mal seizures at home in one day. According to her, he had his first seizure about 2 years ago, had four to five grand mal seizures since that time, and had been taking diphenylhydantoin sodium (Dilantin), 100 mg., t.i.d., and phenobarbital, 30 mg., t.i.d. Approximately 1 month before this episode, Mr. Lawrence lost his job because of lay-offs at his plant and had been unable to find another job. In the last 3 weeks, he had begun to drink progressively more and was drinking about a fifth of whiskey a day until 3 days ago when he abruptly stopped. Upon admission he was quite nervous, and his wife was not certain whether he had taken all of his prescribed medications during the past week. She gave further information to the doctor and nurse, who were particularly interested in the history of the seizures in relation to frequency, usual time of day, characteristics of the attacks, precipitating factors, and presence or absence of aura.

NURSING INTERVENTION

The patient had another grand mal seizure in the emergency room and was admitted for evaluation. The admitting physician called Mrs. Morton, the charge nurse on the neurology division, to tell her of the admission and to order "seizure precautions" for the patient. She immediately prepared the unit by padding the side rails of the bed, lowering the bed to the lowest level, and loosely taping a padded tongue blade to the inside of the top drawer of the bedside table. For sanitary and psychologic reasons, a padded tongue blade is never taped to bedrails or the headboard or left out on the bedside table. In addition to routine equipment for an admission, she obtained a suction machine and catheters, an oral airway (single, for easier suctioning), oxygen equipment, and a flashlight.

The charge nurse in the emergency room notified Mrs. Morton that Mr. Lawrence was on his way to the division. He was sent on a stretcher with side rails up; wrist restraints were also applied since the stretcher was narrow and the side rails were not as high as those on a regular bed. A padded tongue blade was placed under the pillow for accessibility. Portable oxygen equipment was under the stretcher. A licensed practical nurse accompanied the attendant to give care to the patient if needed in transit.

Mr. Lawrence was lethargic from medications given him in the emergency room. Mrs. Morton checked his vital signs, his pupils for size and reaction to light, and the movement of his arms and legs. She positioned him on his side without restraints, raised the padded side rails, and dimmed the room lights. The signal cord was pinned to his hospital gown so that it would be pulled on if he started to move. Since he had required suctioning in the emergency room, she checked his mouth for dentures or partial plates. There were no signs of injury to any part of his body.

A complete neurologic examination was done by the physician, and orders were written stating that the patient was to be on bed rest with side rails up and no restraints. He was to have a lumbar puncture, an electroencephalogram, fasting blood sugar test, and skull X-ray examination. A brain scan was to be scheduled, pending the results of these tests.

About 4 hours after admission, Mr. Lawrence became more alert and was able to sit up in bed to take fluids. He could remember a feeling of "dizziness" before one seizure at home and a beginning awareness of "blacking out" before the others. About an hour later, a nursing assistant supervised him while he smoked a cigarette. Suddenly he dropped the cigarette, his face lost expression, his eyes rolled back, and he uttered a shrill cry. His teeth were not clenched together; so the nursing assistant quickly inserted the padded tongue blade between his back teeth to keep him from biting his tongue. She stayed with Mr. Lawrence, immediately turned on the signal cord, and put the lighted cigarette out. The side rails were still up; so she rolled the bed flat and pulled the curtains around his bed to screen him from the other patient in the room. The clonic phase of this seizure lasted 95 seconds, after which there was a postictal confusional state for approximately 20 minutes.

The registered nurse who was the team leader saw the signal light on and came promptly. All nursing personnel were aware that Mr. Lawrence's seizures were potentially uncontrolled and could occur at any time. The nursing assistant knew that it was important for her or anyone first noting a seizure to stay with the patient for safety reasons, but that an L.P.N. or an R.N. (or a physician if he was readily available) should be called to make careful observations of the nature of the seizure and to give appropriate care if needed. Since restraints may increase convulsive movements or cause injury if strong resistance occurs, they are not indicated during a seizure. Pillows or extra linen are positioned to prevent injury to the patient's head, which might hit the bed during the clonic phase.

The nurse used the following guidelines to record the characteristics of the seizure and the patient's postictal reactions; this information was reported to the doctor:

1. At onset of seizure
   a. Specific part of body involved
   b. Verbal utterance, if any
2. Position of head, body, extremities
   a. At beginning of seizure
   b. After its onset
3. Movements of body
   a. Tonic-clonic phases
   b. Progression of movements
4. Skin color; diaphoresis
5. Respirations (character and rate)
6. Frothing at mouth; teeth clenched
7. Appearance of eyes
   a. Pupillary reaction to light
   b. Deviation of eyes
8. State of consciousness (length of time unconscious)
9. Incontinence of urine and feces
10. Duration of entire attack
11. Postictal phase—duration of this state
    a. State of alertness
    b. Orientation to surroundings
    c. Vital signs
    d. Appearance of eyes
       (1) Pupillary reaction to light
       (2) Deviation of eyes
    e. Recall of aura
    f. Unusual feeling of discomfort in any part of body
    g. Changes in speech
    h. Headache
    i. Injuries, such as tongue-biting

Mr. Lawrence's diagnostic work-up was completed in 3 days. He had no further seizures after those that occurred during the first 24 hours after admission. No cause was identified for the seizure disorder, but it was presumed that withdrawal from alcohol had precipitated the current seizures. By the time of discharge, the seizures were considered under control by medications and seizure precautions were no longer ordered. A tongue blade remained in the patient's bedside table, but the padding on the side rails was no longer necessary. He could be transported to other parts of the hospital in a wheelchair without restraints; he could take a tub bath or shower without supervision and was allowed out of bed as desired. He could smoke without supervision but was cautioned not to smoke in bed. He was to continue the same dosage of diphenylhydantoin sodium (Dilantin) and phenobarbital at home and was to return to the neurology clinic in 1 month. He was given a medical identification card with his medication dosage and a statement that he had a convulsive disorder; he was to carry this in his wallet to provide necessary information in case he had to receive emergency care in a setting where he was not known. Safety precautions were discussed with the patient and his wife, and the nurse taught Mrs. Lawrence what to do to protect her husband from injury when a seizure occurred. Interviews were arranged for Mr. Lawrence to talk with someone at the local vocational rehabilitation service to obtain help in finding suitable employment. The social worker from the neurology division talked to him about where he could seek help for himself in regard to his drinking problem.

CHAPTER 27

A WOMAN SUFFERING A CEREBRAL VASCULAR ACCIDENT

PATRICIA S. BUERGIN AND MARY E. BUSHONG

MEDICAL HISTORY

Mrs. Rogers, an active, 67-year-old retired secretary, was hospitalized after suffering a middle cerebral artery thrombosis. This cerebral vascular accident left her with a dense left hemiparesis and left visual field cut. After 3 days of coma she began to respond, without confusion, and after 3 more days she experienced minimal return of function of her left leg. Over the following period of 8 to 9 weeks, there was slow but progressive return of function in the left leg and return of gross muscular function in the left arm. By the end of 9 weeks, Mrs. Rogers was walking with a straight cane and short leg brace and was wearing a sling on her left arm for support and prevention of subluxation of the left shoulder. The nursing staff succeeded in making her aware of her visual deficit and taught her how to compensate for it.

PSYCHOSOCIAL BACKGROUND

Mrs. Rogers had lived alone in a second story walk-up apartment for 5 years. Although she was making progress during her hospitalization, it was slow enough that she realized she could not return to her independent living situation. Her only son lived in a city 120 miles distant. He was quite concerned for her well-being and told her on one of his visits that he wanted her to come and live with him and his wife. For Mrs. Rogers this meant uprooting herself from the city in which she lived for 67 years, leaving behind all her friends and possessions, and moving to a new city where she knew only her son and daughter-in-law. Where could she meet new friends? What activities could she substitute for those in the past? The social worker discussed Mrs. Rogers' situation with her thoroughly and suggested possible community resources and ideas that could lead to a new way of life. Despite deep emotions over the prospect of making this drastic change in her life pattern, the social worker's interest and support helped Mrs. Rogers express her feelings and accept the alternatives that offered hope for fulfillment in the future. Thus she was able to make the decision to go and live with her son.

NURSING INTERVENTION

Throughout her hospital course, Mrs. Rogers received care and teaching from the interdisciplinary team—occupational therapy, physical therapy, nursing, medicine, and social service. All attempts were made to integrate her abilities toward the goal of self-care. By the time she had made her decision to move to her son's home, she was managing most of her bathing, dressing, and toileting activities independently. The self-care areas in which she still needed assistance, such as putting on the brace, washing her right arm, going up and down stairs, were minimal, but nevertheless present.

It was important for Mrs. Rogers' own self-esteem that she be allowed to perform independently what activities she could, but it was also important that she have assistance for those activities in which she needed it. Arrangements were made through the social worker and the nurse for Mrs. Rogers' son and daughter-in-law to spend an entire day with her, becoming acquainted with the kinds of help she needed, with the areas in which she did not need help, and with the care of the appliances (brace, cane, sling) that she had to use. The nurse who had been working with Mrs. Rogers was assigned to work with the family and instruct them as necessary. Mrs. Rogers' daughter-in-law learned quickly. She was aware of her mother-in-law's desire to be as independent as possible and gave her positive encouragement. After being instructed by the nurse on how to walk with Mrs. Rogers, both the son and daughter-in-law supervised her ambulation, rapidly becoming accustomed to the gait she used and how best to position themselves for her safety.

After both family and patient expressed satisfaction that they would be able to manage at home, arrangements were made—through physical therapy and social service—for the purchase of Mrs. Rogers' own brace and cane. Her son also made plans, with the nurse's guidance, to set up a first-floor bedroom in his home. This would be his mother's room and would be convenient to the first-floor bathroom. The nurse did not think that any other special appliances (such as a hospital bed) would be necessary, and Mr. Rogers agreed. Both physician and nurse conferred about the living arrangements that had been made and the family's ability to manage. Satisfied that the plans were comprehensive, the physician set a discharge date that was acceptable to both patient and family and Mrs. Rogers was discharged 10 weeks after her stroke.

CHAPTER 28

CHANGES IN LIFE-STYLE OF A WOMAN WITH RHEUMATOID ARTHRITIS

CAROLYN BINGHAM DAVIS AND ELLEN HILE DAUGHERTY

MEDICAL HISTORY

Mrs. Bogle, age 44, has had rheumatoid arthritis for the past 4 years. She lived in a two-story house with her husband, a 16-year-old daughter, and a 13-year-old son. A married son, age 21, lived in the same city. During this time, Mrs. Bogle has had intermittent involvement in her right hip and both hands and elbows. Her doctor prescribed enteric-coated aspirin (Ecotrin), 960 mg., with meals and at bedtime with milk; prednisone, 2.5 mg., b.i.d.; range of motion exercises; 1-hour rest periods in the morning and afternoon and 10 hours sleep at night; hot tub baths in the morning and at night; and hydrocollator packs to affected joints p.r.n. She wore bilateral resting splints on her wrists and hand for 6 months prior to her hospitalization.

She worried about taking so many pills every day because of the cost and the influence it might have on her teen-age children "in this age of pill-taking." She kept medicines locked up, since her 1½-year-old grandchild visited frequently. This, however, made it harder for her to remember to take them because the bottles were not in an obvious place. When the dosages were changed, she left a note to herself on the refrigerator door and on the clock radio at her bedside; this helped her remember when medications were due. The doctor gave her a wallet identification card that contained information on her medications; this was especially important since she was on steroids. The doctor also explained that she should not increase or decrease the prednisone without his direction. Occasionally she omitted some of the Ecotrin on days when she felt especially good and took one extra at each dosage time when she had increased pain or stiffness; this was done on her doctor's advice. She watched for gastric problems, ringing in the ears, and any changes in stool color, and reported them to her doctor. An ounce of an antacid or a glass of milk was prescribed for mild gastric upset.

Despite medical treatments and splints, Mrs. Bogle's left hand continued to

165

deviate toward the ulnar side; so she was hospitalized for corrective orthopedic surgery. She also experienced increased pain in her hip and knee joints; so indomethacin (Indocin), 25 mg., b.i.d., was added to her medications and was to be increased to 25 mg., q.i.d., if tolerated.

LABORATORY FINDINGS

During this exacerbation, her erythrocyte sedimentation rate was high (40 mm. in the Wintrobe method) and latex fixation was positive. Other laboratory tests were within normal limits: stool was negative for guaiac; hematocrit was 38 vol.%; white blood count was 7000/ml.

NURSING INTERVENTION

During the hospitalization, nurses and therapists encouraged Mrs. Bogle to tell them about her daily activities and the problems or limitations she encountered at home. The staff were then able to review and discuss simplified or adapted techniques that would enable her to be independent. Once the immediate operative period was over, she practiced adhering to her usual home routine of medications and treatments while still in the hospital setting. When she returned for a medical checkup 6 weeks after discharge, she also had an appointment with the nurse who had been responsible for her care. The following are examples of activities of daily living that Mrs. Bogle was able to work out in joint planning with the nursing team and her family.

Although she is able to continue most of her activities, one of the biggest problems is disciplining herself to allow for the prescribed rest, treatments, medications, and exercises so that she can still have time for household and social activities. She formerly worked part-time as a waitress, but had to give this up because of the physical stresses of irregular hours and long periods of standing and carrying heavy platters.

Mrs. Bogle leaves Ecotrin and milk in a thermos bottle by her bedside so that she can take this at least one-half hour before arising. Just before she gets out of bed she performs range of motion exercises of the prescribed joints slowly five times each. This requires an additional 10 to 15 minutes, and so she sets her clock back to allow sufficient time for this before getting up to prepare breakfast for the family. To save time, she or her daughter sets the table the night before.

Dishwashing is a practical way to apply warm moist heat to the wrists and hands and was resumed as soon as sufficient healing from the surgery occurred. The twice-daily tub baths provide more moist heat to joints, but the humidity in the room makes it hard for Mrs. Bogle to keep her hair-do in place. Because brush rollers are easier for her than are bobby pins, she uses them with plastic stick pins for daily "touch-ups" to her hair. A long-handled back sponge, safety strips in the tub, and handrails on the wall make bathing easier and safer. If her hip or knee involvement becomes worse, other bathroom aids, such as a small stool in the tub and an elevated toilet seat, may be necessary. These high surfaces make rising from a sitting position easier.

Since her husband is at work every weekday with the family car, Mrs. Bogle rides the bus and does some grocery shopping during nonrush hours. At these times, a bus seat is available and minimal lines in the store decrease standing time; this also corresponds to the maximum effectiveness time of her Ecotrin. Familiarity with the store allows preplanned shopping lists to correspond to aisle lay-outs. Buying in small amounts allows use of the express check-out line, and the groceries are less strenuous to carry. Perishable and lightweight foods are purchased on these trips. Heavy items and large quantities are bought during weekend shopping in the car. Both her daughter and her husband help with shopping.

Because her finger and wrist involvement interferes with lifting and certain hand activities, Mrs. Bogle serves buffet style from the stove. She also uses a special lid opener to open screw-topped jars. Since a standard iron is lighter in weight than a steam iron, she sprinkles her clothes before ironing with it. She also sits on a high stool while ironing and preparing food because this position puts less stress on the affected hip and knee joints.

Getting fully dressed every day may be tiring, especially when joints are swollen and painful, but it is important that Mrs. Bogle continue her normal role at home and in her community as much as she can. She avoids buying clothing with small buttons or zippers in the back as well as necklaces and pins with difficult fasteners. She either fastens her brassiere in the front and turns it around or wears a bra slip. Pantyhose also makes dressing easier.

Mrs. Bogle sometimes wakes up in the middle of the night with pain and stiffness and worries when she has to waken her husband to help her turn over in bed or to help her out of bed and to the bathroom. She is able to do these things independently during the day between medications and treatments. The doctor recommended an additional 640 mg. of Ecotrin and milk and a heating pad if she does not want to prepare hydrocollator packs in the night. Mr. Bogle plans to construct blocks to raise the bed to a higher level so that she will have less trouble getting in and out. The firm mattress prevents unnecessary sagging of joints.

Stair-climbing and long periods of standing can be painful for hip and knee joints; so Mrs. Bogle plans activities carefully between the two floors of her home. She keeps milk in a thermos and duplicate supplies of medicines in the upstairs bedroom-bathroom area. Since there is no bathroom on the first floor, she tries to use the toilet when she is upstairs for rest periods and tub baths. She used to be quite active in church and social groups, but has to be more selective now about which ones she attends, since long periods of sitting in meetings, traveling during rush hours, and staying out late at night interfere with rest and treatments. The patient, being a mother of teen-agers, is presented with the special problems of trying to give enough time to the children and their activities. Mrs. Bogle wants to look nice and she wants to maintain an attractive home so that the children can bring their friends to visit. She dusts with the vacuum and mops the floor and the bathtub with long-handled sponges to prevent stooping and kneeling. Some housework is planned for each day, rather than the entire house in one day, and duplicate cleaning supplies are kept on each floor. The family helps with tasks involving heavy lifting or walking.

It has been hard for Mrs. Bogle to learn to accept realistic help. She has always been the one in the family to help others and "keep things going." She does not want to impose on anyone and did not want to be "a cripple" in the eyes of her husband and children. The nurse discussed this with her, emphasizing that she can continue to be active and independent but that she must allow family members and friends to do certain things so that she will have time to follow her medical regime. The family understands that Mrs. Bogle feels better and is more active on some days than others and that it is hard for her to give up some of her very active life. They, too, will need continued support from the interdisciplinary team throughout the chronic course of her illness.

CHAPTER 29

A WOMAN HAVING SURGERY FOR RHEUMATOID ARTHRITIS

ARDITH SUDDUTH AND RUTH BUTLER

MEDICAL HISTORY

Mrs. Alice Manning, a 58-year-old white married woman, was admitted 2 days prior to a scheduled arthrodesis of the right knee. Mrs. Manning was told that she had rheumatoid arthritis when she was 32. She has become progressively more debilitated. Although she has full range of motion of the hip joints bilaterally, she has fairly severe knee joint flexure contractures, thus limiting her mobility. It was hoped that an arthrodesis of the right knee, an artificial ankylosing in the best functional position, would give her a stable, pain-free joint for weight bearing and walking.

She has slight flexure contractures of both elbows and wrists. Because of muscle wasting in the hands, she has only a 50% to 75% grip remaining. She also has slight ulnar drifting in both hands, further decreasing her grip and manual dexterity. Radiographically, all of Mrs. Manning's joints show some arthritic changes.

Mrs. Manning has a history of urinary tract infections, the last one being treated 3 months prior to admission. She also has a history of guaiac positive stools, which were believed to be related to gastric bleeding secondary to large doses of aspirin.

PSYCHOSOCIAL BACKGROUND

Mrs. Manning lives with her husband and 28-year-old daughter on the first floor of a two-story home located on 15 acres of partially cultivated land. Her husband is 62 years of age. He is currently working for a small industrial firm and earns approximately $6,000 a year. He expects to retire at age 65 on a pension of $100 per month plus Social Security benefits. Mrs. Manning is unable to work outside the home. During her hospitalization, she voiced considerable concern about the financial state of their retirement years and the cost of her progressively debilitating illness. Financial concerns were compounded by worry over the 28-year-old daughter who has cerebral palsy manifested by being mentally slow, although she did finish the 6th grade. The daughter is able to stay alone during the day while her mother is in the hospital. Mrs. Manning and her husband have been discussing possible solutions for the care of their daughter when they become unable to care for her in the home. Their other child, also a daughter, is currently working abroad for the United States government. Her achievements are a source of pride for Mrs. Manning.

Mrs. Manning is able to do the laundry and cooking for her family and derives much personal satisfaction in being useful to them. Her husband does the marketing, and her daughter can do simple housekeeping with guidance. Mrs. Manning has been active in the local Catholic church until the past year when walking became much more difficult. She was able to drive a car until approximately 1 year ago.

PREOPERATIVE MEDICAL THERAPY
Medical orders

Indomethacin (Indocin), 25 mg., b.i.d., with meals.

Maalox, 30 ml., p.r.n., with lunch and supper.

Aluminum hydroxide (Amphojel), 30 ml., p.r.n., at breakfast and bedtime. When giving an antacid with medications, make choice according to bowel status; that is, for diarrhea give aluminum hydroxide (Amphojel); for constipation give Maalox.

Darvon, 65 mg., q.3h., p.r.n.

Chloral hydrate, 500 mg., q.h.s., p.r.n.

A.S.A., 960 mg., q.i.d. with meals and h.s. snack.

Skim milk, 120 ml., q.2h., between meals.

Hexachlorophene soap scrub of right leg, groin to ankle, b.i.d., for 10 min.

House diet.

N.P.O. after 10:00 P.M.

Morning of surgery:

Meperidine HCl, 100 mg.   ⎫
Atropine, 0.5 mg.   ⎬ I.M. on call.
                                       ⎭

Laboratory data

ECG, chest X-ray film, RBC, WBC, hematocrit, urine analysis—all within normal limits.

PREOPERATIVE NURSING CARE

DATA	OBJECTIVES	NURSING INTERVENTIONS
First surgical procedure. Her husband cannot take time off from work; her two sisters will come the day of surgery.	Give preoperative instructions after ascertaining what she already knows.	Explain the following to Mrs. Manning: What will happen to her prior to surgery, during surgery, and after surgery; that is, skin preparation with hexachlorophene soap twice a day; N.P.O. after 10:00 P.M.; family should be here by 7:00 A.M., since she is scheduled for surgery at 8:00 A.M. Medication will be given prior to going to the operating room. Intravenous anesthetic will be administered in the operating room. Will awaken with a cast on right leg and I.V. in arm; when awake, will be transferred from recovery room back to the division. Her family may wait on the division for her return from the recovery room; the division secretary will notify family when she has reached the recovery room.
	Teach deep-breathing and leg exercises.	Show how to breathe deeply with diaphragm; have Mrs. Manning repeat process q.i.d. and

Continued.

PREOPERATIVE NURSING CARE —cont'd

DATA	OBJECTIVES	NURSING INTERVENTIONS
		when she thinks of it each day prior to surgery; instruct her to bend left leg as much as possible; instruct in quadriceps-tightening exercises: tighten muscles on thighs and hold for count of 2, and then relax; repeat exercise for each leg q.i.d. and as she thinks of it.
	Teach to void while lying in bed.	Use fracture pan and place it from left side; have Mrs. Manning practice until she can void, using bedpan with ease.
Skin preparation, including shaving and antiseptic scrub, will be done by operating room technician immediately prior to the procedure.	Prepare skin for surgery.	Scrub circumference of right leg with pHiso-Hex from groin to ankle b.i.d. (9:00 A.M., prior to shower, and 8:00 P.M.). Morning of surgery scrub at 6:00 A.M. and wrap leg in sterile legging.
	Morning of surgery prepare for the operating room.	Remove hair pins. Assure oral hygiene. Void—record time and and amount. Tape wedding ring; place other valuables in locked drawer or give to her sisters. Give preanesthetic medication as ordered. Answer any questions she raises. Complete operating room checklist of preparations.

POSTOPERATIVE MEDICAL THERAPY
Medical orders

Meperidine HCl (Demerol), 75 mg., I.M., q.4h., p.r.n., for pain for 48 hours.
2000 ml. 5% dextrose in water at rate of 100 ml./h.
When she is awake, let her take sips of water and advance as tolerated to
1200-calorie diet.
On second postoperative day, resume preoperative medications.
Hydrocollator packs to cervical spine, knees, anterior shoulders, and wrists
for 20 min. in morning.
Physical therapy at 11:00 A.M.
Occupational therapy at 2:00 P.M.

Laboratory data

Urinalysis, remained within normal limits.
Stool for guaiac, positive on fourth and fifth postoperative days, negative
thereafter.

IMMEDIATE POSTOPERATIVE NURSING CARE
(FIRST 24 HOURS)

DATA	OBJECTIVES	NURSING INTERVENTIONS
Mrs. Manning's BP was 120/80 immediately upon her return and rose to 130/80 where it remained; her BP prior to surgery was 140/78.	Monitor vital signs for indications of hemorrhage or shock.	Hospital routine was followed: 1. BP and pulse q.15-min. × 4, q.30min. × 4, q.1h. × 4, then q.4h. 2. Temperature q.4h.; after 24 hours postoperatively, her BP and T.P.R. were monitored q.i.d.; on the fourth postoperative day, vital signs were checked b.i.d.
Cast applied from groin to ankle.	Monitor right toes for signs of circulatory impairment.	Check toes q.1h. for signs of circulatory embarrassment: color, capillary refill, temperature, sensation of pain or prickling.

Continued.

IMMEDIATE POSTOPERATIVE NURSING CARE
(FIRST 24 HOURS)—cont'd

DATA	OBJECTIVES	NURSING INTERVENTIONS
Balanced suspension traction applied to bed.	Facilitate circulation to right leg.	Keep right leg elevated 4 to 6 inches in balanced suspension traction free from pillows; have her perform quadriceps tightening q.1h. as she is able.
	Facilitate general circulation.	Leg exercises to left leg: 1. Quadriceps tightening 2. Leg bending to continue throughout hospitalization
	Promote respiratory O_2-CO_2 exchange.	Deep breathing and coughing q.1h. until h.s.; then, q.4h. when vital signs checked; continue throughout hospitalization.
	Promote rest and comfort.	Keep right leg elevated. Give meperidine HCl I.M., q.4h., p.r.n. for pain for 24 hours; then Darvon Compound, 65 mg., orally q.4h., p.r.n. Help to change positions q.1h., coordinate with monitoring vital signs to allow rest periods.
N.P.O. since 10:00 P.M. night before surgery. 250 ml. blood loss in surgery not replaced.	Maintain adequate fluid intake.	Check I.V. each time in room; keep running at 100 ml./h. Offer sips of water as soon as awake.
	Begin meeting nutritional needs of body.	Order full liquid diet for breakfast and soft diet for lunch and supper.
	Promote urinary elimination.	Offer bedpan by 3:00 P.M.; if unable to void, offer bedpan q.½h. until she voids.

IMMEDIATE POSTOPERATIVE NURSING CARE
(FIRST 24 HOURS)—cont'd

DATA	OBJECTIVES	NURSING INTERVENTIONS
		Try running water in sink, warming bedpan, etc., to facilitate voiding.
Mrs. Manning was able to void by 4:00 P.M. History of bladder infections.		Offer fluids frequently.

POSTOPERATIVE NURSING CARE

Mrs. Manning had an uneventful immediate postoperative recovery. On her first postoperative day, the following care plan was adopted and continually modified until her discharge from the hospital on her twentieth postoperative day. She was hospitalized for this period of time so that she could learn to care for herself with the cast on and until she could learn exercises in physical therapy to strengthen her shoulder and arm muscles and to improve and maintain hand function.

NURSING CARE PLAN

DATA	OBJECTIVES	NURSING INTERVENTIONS
Hydrocollator packs 20 min. before physical therapy; heat reduces morning joint stiffness of arthritis.	Facilitate muscle relaxation and comfort.	Apply six layers of towel between packs and skin. Check after 5 min. for redness, heat, and feeling of being too hot; place another towel if necessary between packs and skin.
Mrs. Manning receives great deal of comfort from packs, which also increases her ability to care for herself.		Have Mrs. Manning lie on her back; place one hydrocollator pack on each shoulder, knee, and wrist; after 20 min. turn to left side and place two hydrocollator packs to cervical spine.

Continued.

NURSING CARE PLAN—cont'd

DATA	OBJECTIVES	NURSING INTERVENTIONS
Mrs. Manning has some discomfort in her right leg and her arthritic joints; she has a tendency to allow others to do whatever they are willing to do for her.	Maintain good hygiene; promote independence in as many areas of self care as possible.	Place oral hygiene articles on overbed table; after completion of oral hygiene, place basin of bath water on overbed table with 2 capfuls of bath oil, soap, and towels. Wash back and buttocks. Inspect for signs of increased pressure—redness, tissue breakdown.
Likes lotion and her own powder for back care. Can bathe self except for back and toes of right foot.		Use hospital lotion and her powder for back care. Wash between toes of right leg with small cotton swabs; dry carefully; place small pieces of cotton between each toe.
	Promote circulation in right leg.	Keep leg elevated. In wheelchair, elevate right leg and tie casted leg to wheelchair leg with Ace wrap. Check toes for color, capillary fill, temperature; record. Check leg and cast for signs of infection or drainage—increased pain, odor, drainage on cast.
No weight bearing on right leg. At first, needed one person to hold cast and one person to assist her into wheelchair; after first week, needed only one person to hold cast, and she could transfer herself into wheelchair.	Transfer from bed to wheelchair.	Uses two persons first week; later, one person to hold cast; use following procedure: Remove right arm of wheelchair. Place wheelchair lengthwise at left side of bed.

NURSING CARE PLAN—cont'd

DATA	OBJECTIVES	NURSING INTERVENTIONS
		Place bed flat. Have Mrs. Manning scoot to edge of bed. Have her sit up on edge of bed, nurse supporting cast. Left foot on floor; pivot on left foot into chair. Replace arm on chair. Attach weight on back of chair for balance.
History of urinary tract infections.	Promote urinary elimination.	Offer fluids often during day; push fluids to 2500 ml. daily; likes coffee, tea, iced water, diet cola. Offer to assist onto commode or bedpan q.2h.
	Prevent urinary tract infections.	Teach to wipe self from front to back. Teach perineal care with aseptic wipe after each voiding.
Mrs. Manning likes to void in private and to care for herself privately.		Be sure privacy maintained during toileting. Observe urine for amount, color, odor. Report any deviations from normal.
Stool for guaiac daily. Problems with constipation during hospitalization. Guaiac positive on third and fourth postoperative days. Uses commode daily for B.M.	Promote bowel elimination.	Give Maalox as antacid on days stools are hard. Alternate Maalox with aluminum hydroxide (Amphojel) to maintain stools. Send stool for guaiac. Observe stools for bleeding, color, and consistency. Record character of stool.

Continued.

NURSING CARE PLAN—cont'd

DATA	OBJECTIVES	NURSING INTERVENTIONS
Aspirin, 960 mg., q.i.d.; aspirin is an ulcerogenic drug.	Reduce gastrointestinal irritation.	Give aspirin with meals and antacid. Give 120 ml. of skim milk q.2h. when awake (8:00 A.M.–10:00 P.M.)
Mrs. Manning is 5 feet, 2 inches tall and weighs 140 lb. Weight reduction necessary to reduce stress on weight-bearing joints. 1200-calorie diet. Dietitian at first spent time each day with Mrs. Manning; later, only once a week.	Maintain nutritional intake to meet metabolic needs.	Arrange for dietitian to see Mrs. Manning about 1200-calorie diet, including 120 ml. of skim milk q.2h.
Mrs. Manning will be in wheelchair for approximately 6 weeks before cast removed.		Plan a kitchen evaluation with occupational therapy. O.T. will arrange for work-saving devices.
Preparing food is one way Mrs. Manning feels useful and important to her family.		Allow her to discuss her feelings about food preparation and her role in the family.
28-year-old daughter is overweight and has hypertension.		Help her see how she can prepare low-calorie foods that are palatable and appealing and that meet the nutritional needs of her family.
Mrs. Manning has a progressively debilitating illness.	Help her accept the optimum possible goals in the light of physical limitations.	Allow to do as much for herself as possible. Help her make a realistic plan for activities of daily living, including rest periods between activities.
Husband seems to have a good understanding of his wife's illness and is willing to cooperate in her care as needed.		Help her involve her family in these plans. Help her adjust to her changing body image by showing her she is accepted as she is.

NURSING CARE PLAN—cont'd

DATA	OBJECTIVES	NURSING INTERVENTIONS
Mrs. Manning has become progressively more unable to leave home and mingle with others.		Help her plan ways to be with others; that is, arrange with church ladies' group to pick her up and take her to a meeting.
She was active in church circle until 1 year ago.		
She has feelings of insecurity, helplessness, and anxiety and at times tends to withdraw, especially from strangers.	Help her identify and accept positive and negative expressions, feelings, and reactions.	Listen to her. Help her understand that the nurse is genuinely interested in her, her concerns, and her progress.
Usually responds warmly to strangers (nurse, visitors, patients) in 10 to 15 min.	Keep the lines of verbal and nonverbal communication open between nurse and Mrs. Manning and Mrs. Manning and others.	Follow her routine when new to her care. Give her time to get to know nurse.
Concerned about financial status. Concerned about care of daughter in distant future.		Allow her to discuss her financial concerns and her concerns about long-term care of her daughter. Arrange for social worker to talk with her for possible help with these problems: perhaps there are agencies and programs where she could qualify for some sort of assistance; perhaps there are agencies to help plan the care for her daughter.
	Plan for immediate home going.	Help her arrange for a wheelchair. Discuss ways to take bed bath or a bath at sink at home. (Kitchen planning done by occupational therapy.)

Continued.

NURSING CARE PLAN—cont'd

DATA	OBJECTIVES	NURSING INTERVENTIONS
		Help plan for activities of living with a cast on leg and no weight bearing on that leg. Help plan ways daughter can assist in household activities and care.

Mrs. Manning liked a set routine for her personal care and daily activities; therefore the following schedule was set up for her:

DATA	SCHEDULE
	Morning:
	7:45, Wash for breakfast.
	8:00, Breakfast.
	8:30, Hydrocollator packs to knees, shoulder, and wrists.
	8:40, Packs off.
	8:50-9:10, Place packs on cervical spine.
Bathroom too small for wheelchair.	9:15, Up on bedpan or commode for B.M.
	9:30-9:45, Rest.
	9:45, Bath articles set up.
	10:00, Nurse wash back and toes of right foot.
	10:15, Comb hair; put on makeup.
	10:30, Up in wheelchair and out in hall to socialize with other patients.
	11:00, To physical therapy.
	Afternoon:
	12:00, Return from physical therapy to dining room for lunch.
	1:00-2:00, To bed for rest period.
	2:15, Occupational therapy.
	3:15, Return; socialize with others.
	4:00-5:00, To bed for rest period.
	5:00, Up in wheelchair for supper.
	5:15, Wash at sink for supper.
	5:30, Supper.
	6:30, Commode; to bed.
	7:00, Family and friends sometimes visit.
Always stays up until 11:00-11:30 P.M. at home.	8:00-11:00, Relaxes watching T.V.

Mrs. Manning was discharged to her home with her right leg in a cast and she was unable to bear weight on it. Her husband rented a wheelchair for the 6 weeks she was at home. She was then readmitted to the hospital for 10 days, at which time her cast was removed and she participated in an active physical therapy program, including weight bearing on the right leg and walking with a cane. When Mrs. Manning went home, she was able to walk for short distances (one-half to one block) and could manage her personal care and household duties.

CHAPTER 30

AN ADOLESCENT BOY WITH PROGRESSIVE SCOLIOSIS

DONNA J. KUKLO

MEDICAL HISTORY AND PSYCHOSOCIAL BACKGROUND

Glen, a 13-year-old boy, looked for all the world like a little hunchbacked old man. He listed to the left side and dragged his left leg behind him and was so twisted and bent that his height was less than 5 feet. His face, though, was round and smiling and had an impish look on it. His body was rotund with fat, but lacked the muscle tone of a normal teen-ager.

Glen was the youngest of three children. His sister, age 26, was married and had two small children. His 22-year-old brother was in the Army serving in Southeast Asia. Glen talked a good deal about his mother and his brother and sister, but infrequently mentioned his father. He would explain that his father did not come to visit him because he worked "the afternoon shift" during the week and did not like to drive so far for such short visits. The father did bring Glen's mother to the city on Sundays so that she could stay at her sister's home and be in town to visit Glen each day. He came to take her home each Friday evening. Glen's tone of voice seemed to indicate that his father was not happy over the inconvenience of Glen's present hospitalization.

The boy spoke with affection of the little lake community, 60 miles away, in which he lives, referring to it as a quiet and restful place where life centers around the family and not on social activities. The houses are spread out around the lake. The people live there all year long, and there seems to be a spirit of neighborliness within the community.

The hospital was not new to Glen. At 21 months of age he developed polio and spent the following 3 years in and out of a hospital located 15 miles away from his home. The muscles of all four extremities as well as his trunk and intercostal muscles were involved. During these early hospitalizations, he spent most of the time in a respirator or in a rocking bed.

When he was 5 years old, Glen was placed in long-leg braces so that he could be more mobile. He regained most of the strength in his arm muscles, but his trunk and leg muscles remained weak. At this time, he was able to walk for short periods on even surfaces with the aid of braces, but had difficulty in managing his balance on uneven ground outdoors.

The onset of structural paralytic scoliosis came when Glen was 8 years old. Because of the inadequacy of his trunk musculature, the vertebral column eventually collapsed and became fixed in severe deformity. The easy fatigability that he experienced at this time probably resulted from his being in an erect position without trunk support. In an effort to keep the curvature from becoming worse, he was placed in a Milwaukee brace. An arthrodesis of the left foot was done to correct a valgus deformity.

Glen entered the hospital this time to have a spinal fusion. His scoliosis had progressed to the point of interfering drastically with his vital capacity. Some respiratory muscle paralysis often accompanies extensive weakness of trunk musculature. The method of cast application usually used to correct scoliosis was not advisable in Glen's case, since the cast would produce pressure on his chest wall, further interfering with proper ventilation. If a spinal fusion was to be done, there would have to be some method for keeping his spinal column immobile after the fusion while at the same time not compromising his vital capacity. It was decided that Glen would be put in halo traction with a frame.

The halo frame provided immobilization of the head and neck and permitted longitudinal traction to stretch and straighten the curvature. Glen had the halo frame applied 3 weeks prior to the spinal fusion. Besides the halo attachment to the head, the appliance also included a Milwaukee brace and bilateral leg casts.

PREOPERATIVE NURSING CARE OBJECTIVES

The major objectives for Glen at this time were the following:

1. *To maintain adequate pulmonary ventilation.* It was particularly important to look for signs and symptoms of hypoventilation and hyperventilation. Glen's vital capacity before application of the halo frame was 62% of his predicted normal value. After application, it was 69%. Respiratory assistive equipment must be available for emergency use, if vital capacity falls below 60%.

2. *To teach the procedure of coughing and deep breathing.* Most patients with respiratory deficit have difficulty coughing. Physical therapy personnel taught Glen how to cough and breathe deeply. The nursing staff taught him to use the IPPB machine and encouraged him to practice his coughing and deep-breathing exercises every 2 hours.

3. *To maintain skin integrity.* Turning was essential not only to ventilate his

lungs, but also to provide a shift in body weight to prevent development of pressure areas. Glen could only be placed supine or on his side. Because of the construction of the apparatus, the heels and the skin under the pelvic band were subject to pressure. Folded bath blankets were placed under the ankles to alleviate heel pressure. The skin under the pelvic band was observed for signs of irritation, especially when the band became loose as Glen moved. The orthopedist readjusted the pelvic girdle periodically.

4. *To prevent infection of the skin surrounding the screws that held the halo in place.* The halo is attached to the external cortex of the cranium by two anterior and two posterior screws. The skin at these sites is liable to become inflamed and to drain serous fluid. A crust forms when the fluid dries. Daily cleaning of the skin surrounding the screws helps prevent infection.

5. *To teach Glen to clean these areas.* He became quite independent in carrying out the task with a mirror and long-stemmed cotton swabs. He boasted of the fact that not one of the screw attachment areas became infected.

6. *To maintain alignment of legs.* The bilateral leg casts were attached by hooks to the frame to maintain tension on the lower extremities. To prevent internal and external rotation of Glen's legs when he was supine, the nurse tied the ankles of the casts to the frame in a neutral position. While he lay on his side and during turning, pillows were placed between his legs to maintain proper leg alignment.

7. *To maintain muscle strength of upper extremities.* Inactivity and bed rest result in muscular atrophy. Passive arm exercises were administered each morning at bathtime. Glen provided active exercise when he cared for the skin around the screw attachments, when he ate, when he brushed his teeth, and when he washed his face and arms.

8. *To maintain adequate nutrition and elimination.* Since Glen was normally not an active boy, being restricted to the frame did not bring about much change in his eating and elimination patterns. He had little difficulty in feeding himself, and he enjoyed doing this independently. He required assistance only in cutting meat and in opening milk cartons. He was able to take fluids on his own when these were placed within reach. He adjusted well to the regular hospital diet. He was given a stool softener each day to prevent constipation.

9. *To provide privacy.* Glen was at the age when boys are normally very aware of their bodies and are often shy about having another person in the room when they are bathing or toileting. He manifested concern about having someone place the urinal for him when he needed to urinate. When his mother was in the room, he preferred that she do this for him, rather than one of the younger nurses.

10. *To provide diversion that would be intellectually stimulating and would exercise his arms.* Glen was unable to attend regular school; he had a tutor at home. He was an avid reader and was able to keep up with his classes; he surpassed his peers in English and history. At home he spent most of his time reading, watching television, or playing cards. Miss Jay, a junior nursing student, was able to obtain a pair of prism glasses for him from Library Services so that he could watch television in the hospital. She asked the occupational therapist to provide a project for him that would help to exercise his upper extremities. The therapist visited him weekly and gave him materials for making wallets, key cases, etc.

11. *To provide information during the preoperative period.* Glen was at an age of curiosity and inquisitiveness. He was intensely interested in details of the surgical procedure and in things that happen in the intensive care unit. The orthopedist explained the purpose of the halo frame and the casts; he described the spinal fusion procedures. Glen sought additional help from the nurses. He asked, "How will the doctor connect the (bone) pieces?" Miss Jay made a sketch of two vertebrae to show him how the iliac bone chips fit between the vertebrae. Additional explanation, that these pieces grow together like skin after being cut, helped him to understand how a spinal column becomes solid. When Miss Jay discussed postoperative care, Glen's mother was present. She and Glen knew that he would spend at least one night in the surgical intensive care unit. They asked many questions about visiting hours, the physical plan of the unit, and the kinds of patients that would be there. In addition, Miss Jay tried to prepare them for the variety of machines that they might see.

Miss Jay reminded Glen about the need to cough and deep-breathe periodically after surgery. She also acquainted him with the possibility that he might awaken in a mist tent and remain in it for several days after surgery. Glen seemed to understand his need for adequate ventilation. He remembered what he had been taught about turning, coughing, and deep-breathing, and said, "I've got to do this to get the junk out of my lungs, so I won't get pneumonia again."

POSTOPERATIVE CARE AND ADJUSTMENT

During surgery the orthopedist decided that a two-stage fusion was required because of marked blood loss. The halo apparatus was replaced; femoral traction and a posterior body cast were also used to maintain body alignment. The surgeon thought that the half shell cast would provide better spine immobilization when Glen was turned.

Immediately after surgery, Glen's hematocrit was 24 vol.%; after two blood transfusions, it rose to 33 vol.%. Because of the blood loss and the danger of pulmonary complications, Glen remained in the intensive care unit for 3 days.

When he returned to the private room that he had occupied previously, the nursing care objectives were essentially the same as they had been before the operation. Adequate pulmonary ventilation was still of prime importance. He remained in a mist tent for 4 more days to assist in raising secretions. Although patients who undergo spinal fusions suffer varying degrees of pain postoperatively, by the time Glen returned to his own room, he had minimal discomfort and required little analgesia. After 8 days, the sutures were removed and the half-shell cast was replaced by the Milwaukee brace.

Once the acute stage of his illness was over, he became more and more interested in plans for going to a rehabilitation hospital for children. Miss Jay suggested that he and his mother keep a pad at his bedside to jot down questions. Both were concerned about the environment of the rehabilitation hospital. Within 2 days, the list of questions grew to two pages: "Where is it located? Will Glen be in a room with other children? What kind of deformities do the others have? Will Glen be with children his own age? Are there provisions for continuing his schooling?" Miss Jay sought answers from several resource persons. Finally she visited the rehabilitation unit to obtain first-hand information that others had not been able to provide.

Throughout Glen's hospitalization there were numerous occasions when Miss Jay identified his need for more information. The environment for teaching is important if one hopes to be effective. Conditions for teaching Glen were ideal. He was a person who related well to peers and adults; he freely verbalized what was on his mind. Since he was in a private room and was immobilized, Miss Jay had an eager learner in surroundings that were free from distractions.

The day of Glen's discharge brought forth mixed emotions. For Glen and his mother, it meant leaving familiar surroundings where his needs were known and readily met. For the staff, it meant the loss of a very pleasant young man with strength of character and courage. Miss Jay summed her feelings when she said, "I feel personal satisfaction in having been a part of Phase I of the plan to help Glen become a straighter, taller young man."

REFERENCES

Barnes, K.: Halo traction, Amer. J. Nurs. 69:1933-1937, Sept. 1969.

Boegli, E. H., and Steele, M. S.: Scoliosis: spinal instrumentation and fusion, Amer. J. Nurs. 68:2399-2403, Nov. 1968.

Ferguson, A., Jr.: Orthopedic surgery in infancy and childhood, ed. 3, Baltimore, 1968, The Williams & Wilkins Co.

Jordan, V., Ohara, Y. L., Smith, M., and Townsley, J. A.: Halo body cast and spinal fusion, Amer. J. Nurs. 63:77-80, Aug. 1963.

Roberts, J. M.: New development in orthopedic surgery—scoliosis, Nurs. Clin. N. Amer. 2:385-386, Sept. 1967.

CHAPTER 31

REHABILITATION OF A MAN WITH A FRACTURED FEMUR

PATRICIA S. BUERGIN AND MARY E. BUSHONG

MEDICAL HISTORY

Mr. Kingman is a 75-year-old gentleman who, until his hospitalization, had been living in a two-room apartment in his daughter's home. Aside from having meals provided, he was able to manage all other activities of daily living. One night, while walking to the bathroom, he fell and suffered an intertrochanteric fracture of the left femur. He was admitted to the hospital, and the next day he was treated by open reduction and internal fixation of the femur with a Smith-Petersen nail and Thornton plate.

NURSING INTERVENTION

The rehabilitation goal for Mr. Kingman was to assist him in regaining his former level of independence. One major emphasis in achieving this goal was the process of reambulation. This process began in the immediate postoperative period. To avoid displacement of the nail while he was lying in bed, the nurse positioned Mr. Kingman with pillows or trochanter rolls as necessary to maintain his hip in a neutral position (avoiding both internal and external rotation). To maintain both muscle tone and circulation in the operated leg, Mr. Kingman was taught to do quadriceps setting, as well as dorsiflexion and plantar flexion exercises. He was also encouraged to do active range of motion exercises with the unoperated leg and to involve that leg in such activities as helping to push himself up in bed.

On the day after surgery, the nurse helped Mr. Kingman sit on the edge of his Hi-Lo bed (in low position) with his operated leg elevated in a chair to prevent edema. He was positioned in such a fashion that his foot on the unoperated side rested squarely on the floor. To strengthen his unoperated leg, he was then asked to successively wiggle his toes, press his foot against the floor, and raise his leg straight out. To help himself to the sitting position and to strengthen his triceps, Mr. Kingman was encouraged to use his arms and hands to push against the bed. He was asked to do all these exercises at least three times a day.

On the third postoperative day the nurse, according to the doctor's order, helped the patient transfer into a wheelchair. Care was taken that he did not bear weight on his operated leg. He was encouraged on this and successive transfers to use his hands and arms as much as possible. He was taught to push against the bed to help himself stand and then to transfer his hands to the arms of his locked wheelchair and lower himself. While in the wheelchair, as while sitting on the edge of the bed, his operated leg was kept elevated at hip level.

One week after surgery, Mr. Kingman began ambulation in parallel bars, bearing weight only on his unoperated leg. These beginning ambulation measures were taught and supervised by a physical therapist. While he was ambulating, Ace wraps were used to prevent dependent edema in his operated leg. Within 4 days Mr. Kingman had progressed to the point of being able to use a walker with close supervision by the nursing staff. Now he was able to put his ambulating skills to functional use on his division, employing the walker to go short distances from bed to bathroom. As his skills and endurance increased, he was expected to walk longer distances. Within 3 weeks he no longer needed to use the wheelchair. During this 3-week period the nurse had also taught him how to safely get on and off a chair, the bed, and the toilet, to be aware of and safely maneuver around obstacles, and to walk on carpeting.

Mr. Kingman's daughter visited her father frequently during his hospital stay and was kept abreast of his progress. When he had reached the point of using a walker independently, the nurse encouraged the daughter to spend a morning with him. The opportunity to see how well he could care for himself and move around made her more comfortable about his returning to her home. Five weeks after surgery, Mr. Kingman was discharged from the hospital to be followed by his physician.

CORRELATION OF PATIENT CARE STUDIES WITH

MEDICAL-SURGICAL NURSING

Chapter in Medical-Surgical Nursing	1	2	3	4	5	6	7	8	9	10	11	12	1.
1 Patient and nurse	X	X			X								
2 Age factor	X	X	X	X	X	X	X	X	X	X	X	X	X
3 Body defenses													
4 Homeostatic state													X
5 Nutrition													X
6 Personality disorders			X										
7 Pain	X												
8 Incontinence				X									
9 Unconsciousness				X									
10 Surgical treatment	X				X						X		
11 Plastic surgery	X												
12 Special continuing care				X									
14 Malignant disease	X	X				X							
16 Cardiac disease							X	X	X	X	X		X
17 Peripheral vascular disease												X	
18 Blood dyscrasias						X							
19 Urinary system disease													X
20 Reproductive system disease													
21 Pulmonary disease						X					X		
23 Disease of teeth and mouth													
24 Gastrointestinal disease	X												
25 Liver disease													
26 Endocrine disease												X	
28 Burns													
29 Disease of breast													
30 Eye disease													
31 Neurologic disease			X										
32 Disease of joints and connective tissues				X									
33 Fractures													

apter in **Patient Care Studies**

14	15	16	17	18	19	20	21	22	23	24	25	26	27	28	29	30	31
X	X	X	X	X	X	X	X	X	X	X	X	X	X	X	X	X	X
							X										
							X										
X				X	X	X											
					X	X						X					
				X					X								
			X	X				X	X						X	X	
X																	
X																	
	X	X															
						X											
			X														
				X	X												
						X											
							X										
								X									
									X								
										X	X	X	X				
														X	X	X	
																	X

162

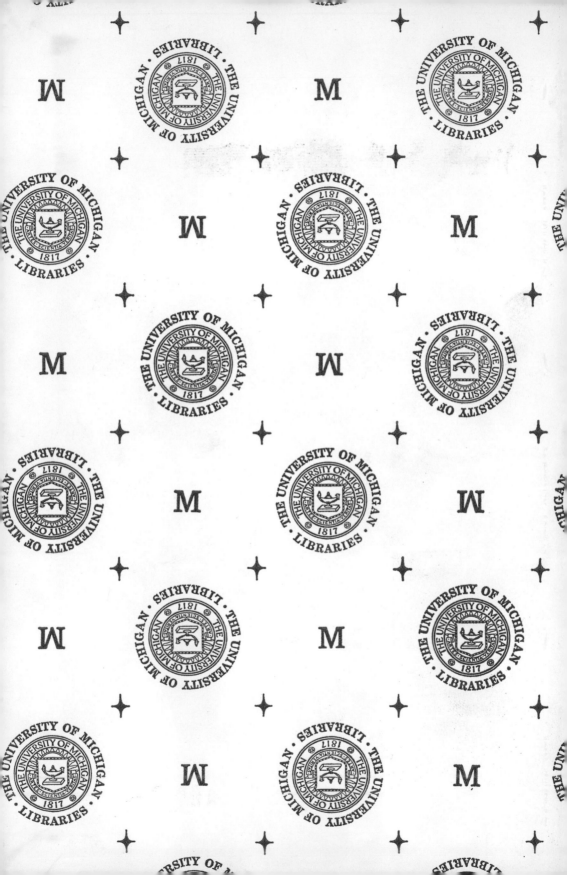